How organisations measure success

How organisations measure success

The use of performance indicators in government

Neil Carter, Rudolf Klein and Patricia Day

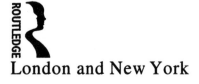

London and New York

First published in 1992
First published in paperback in 1995
by Routledge
11 New Fetter Lane, London EC4P 4EE

Simultaneously published in the USA and Canada
by Routledge
29 West 35th Street, New York, NY 10001

Reprinted in 1993

Typeset by
NWL Editorial Services, Langport, Somerset

Printed and bound in Great Britain by
Mackays of Chatham PLC, Chatham, Kent

British Library Cataloguing in Publication Data
Carter, Neil
 How organisations measure success: the use of performance
 indicators in government.
 1. Great Britain. Organisations. Performance. Assessment
 I. Title II. Klein, Rudolf *1930–* III. Day, Patricia *1940–*
 354.94101

Library of Congress Cataloging in Publication Data
Carter, Neil, 1958–
 How organisations measure success: the use of performance
 indicators in government/Neil Carter, Rudolf Klein, and
 Patricia Day.
 p. cm.
 Includes bibliographical references.
 1. Administrative agencies – Great Britain – Evaluation –
 Case studies. 2. Executive departments – Great Britain –
 Evaluation – Case studies. 3. Government productivity –
 Great Britain – Case studies. 4. Industrial productivity –
 Great Britain – Case studies. I. Klein, Rudolf.
 II. Day, Patricia. III. Title.
 JN318.C37 1991
 354.4107′6 – dc20   91–9120
                                         CIP

ISBN 0–415–04195–3 (hbk)
ISBN 0–415–11912–X (pbk)

Contents

List of tables   vi
List of abbreviations   vii
Introduction   1

1 **Revolution or resurrection? The history of a concept**   5

2 **Models, measures, and muddles: organisational and
   conceptual dimensions of performance indicators**   25

3 **The criminal justice system: police, courts, and prisons**   52

4 **The welfare system: Social Security and the
   National Health Service**   89

5 **The private sector: banks, building societies, and
   retail stores**   118

6 **Managing monopolies: railways, water, and airports**   138

7 **Performance indicators in the 1990s: tools for managing
   political and administrative change**   165

References   184
Name index   192
Subject index   194

Tables

2.1 Organisational dimensions   34
2.2 A selection of alternative input–output models   36
3.1 Notifiable offences recorded and cleared up   56
3.2 Crown Court: committals for trial – average waiting time (in weeks) of defendants dealt with 1983–4 to 1988–9 (England and Wales)   69
3.3 Crown Court: average hours sat per day 1984–5 to 1988–9 (England and Wales)   69
3.4 County Court: the percentage of processes taking longer than five days to issue and dispatch   71
3.5 Average weekly hours of inmate activity delivered per inmate and average numbers of inmates involved in regime activities: April–September 1989   87
4.1 Social Security performance indicators: clearance times (in days)   92
4.2 Social Security performance indicators: error rates (percentage of payments incorrect)   93
4.3 Clearance times (in days) 1986–7   94
4.4 Targets for the Social Security regional organisation   97
4.5 Quality of service statistics 1988–9   100
4.6 Quality Assessment Package 1989–90   101
4.7 Selected National Health Service performance indicators   110
6.1 British Rail performance indicators: a selection showing the performance of the total business and of the InterCity sector   146
6.2 Rail passenger quality of service objectives – 1987   147
6.3 Classification of rivers and canals   156
6.4 BAA financial performance indicators   162
7.1 Characteristics of performance indicators in the case studies   168
7.2 Use of performance indicators in the case studies   169

Abbreviations

APH	Articles per hour
BAA	British Airports Authority
BR(B)	British Railways (Board)
CIPFA	Chartered Institute of Public Finance and Accountancy
CTCC	Central Transport Consultative Committee
DES	Department of Education and Science
DoE	Department of the Environment
DHSS	Department of Health and Social Security
DSS	Department of Social Security
FMI	Financial Management Initiative
HSR	High Street Retailer
LCD	Lord Chancellor's Department
LEA	local education authority
MBO	Management by Objectives
MINIS	Management Information Systems for Ministers
MMC	Mergers and Monopolies Commission
NAO	National Audit Office
NHS	National Health Service
PAR	Programme Analysis and Review
PBO	Policing by Objectives
PI	Performance Indicator
PPBS	Planning, Programming, Budgeting System
PR	Performance Ratio
QAP	Quality Assessment Package
WAA	Water Authorities Association

Introduction

In the 1980s the Thatcher Administration set out to transform the management and style of government. Previous Administrations had set out with the same ambition; none was able to pursue it with such persistence for so long. The Whitehall of the 1990s clearly bears the imprint, and the scars, of the efforts made to ensure that it will be very different from the Whitehall that Mrs Thatcher inherited in 1979. It is a change that goes beyond the introduction of new techniques or the re-drawing of the boundary between the public and the private sectors. It reflects also a challenge to some of the traditional values of the civil service. It demands that the mandarin should be reborn as a manager. It emphasises drive and energy rather than the avoidance of mistakes; it requires loyalty to Ministers and their political goals rather than to some notion of the public goods defined by the civil service. Its vocabulary stresses value for money, efficiency, decentralisation, and accountability. Above all, it represents a determination to change the culture of government.

It remains to be seen how much of Mrs Thatcher's cultural revolution will survive her period in office. To the extent that it reflects a wider transformation in society as a whole, it seems probable that it will. It is unlikely that the civil service will ever again fit comfortably into an establishmentarian mould that has cracked. It is equally unlikely that Whitehall will ever be able to ignore the transformation wrought by information technology in all large organisations. Above all, it is highly implausible that any government will throw away the new tools of management that were developed in the 1980s.

Hence the relevance for the 1990s of this study of the way in which performance indicators (PIs) were developed in the 1980s. Performance indicators were only one element in the overall strategy of making evaluation a feature of the new Whitehall structure. But they were an essential part. If there is to be value for money, then the activities and outputs of government have to be measured; if there is to be more accountability, then there has to be an accepted currency of evaluation; if there is to be decentralisation, and blocks of work are to be hived off without loss of control, then there has to be a way of assessing performance. So it is not surprising that the Prime Minister decreed in the 1982 Financial Management Initiative (FMI) – the manifesto of the revolution – that a thousand PIs should flourish, and that ever since they have indeed multiplied throughout Whitehall. The evolution of the PI system therefore provides an insight into the whole process of change in British Government.

For creating a system of PIs is not just a technical exercise, although it may be seen as such. It raises some fundamental questions of governance. What counts as good performance? How do we define the various dimensions of performance, and what should be the currencies of evaluation embodied in any system? Who determines what is good performance, and who is the audience for PIs? Are PIs tools of control in hierarchic organisations, are they instruments of managerial self-examination or are they devices for preserving accountability while decentralising responsibility? Are they designed for Ministers, for Parliament, for managers, for service users, or for the population at large? In short, to study the evolution of PIs in British Government is to gain an insight into organisational politics and values, and the power of different organisational actors such as the medical profession or the police. It is also to illuminate the conceptual and methodological problems involved in designing new tools of government; one of the reasons why the experience of the 1980s is still highly relevant for the 1990s is that the design task is far from complete (just as one of the reasons why the 1980s exercise was only half successful was that while the concept of PIs was a child of the 1960s, it had suffered from arrested development).

This study addresses these and other issues in a series of case studies of the design and implementation of PI systems in a variety of organisational settings. First, it analyses the way in which different government departments and public services have implemented the PI strategy of making organisational self-evaluation part of the Whitehall culture. Second, and more briefly, it looks at the way in which a variety of private sector organisations have set about the same task. In adopting such a comparative strategy of inquiry, we wanted to test the conventional wisdom that there is some particular quality about the public sector – some Platonic essence of 'publicness' – which makes transplanting techniques from the private sector inappropriate or difficult. Instead, we started from the assumption that, taking the case of PIs, the problems of introducing and developing new techniques might also reflect specific organisational characteristics cutting across the public–private divide. Accordingly our case studies were chosen in order to study the evolution of PI systems in contrasting organisational environments: we explored, for example, whether social security might have more in common with a bank than with the National Health Service (NHS) or a supermarket. For if there is to be a cross-sector learning, if there are to be successful transplants of ideas and techniques, it is essential that the donor should be matched accurately to the recipient.

Our research strategy therefore required us to look at a wide range of organisations, although we make no attempt to deal with them all at the same length or in the same depth. The benefit of such an approach is, in our view, that it allows more insights to be generated than if the inquiry had been confined to either the public or to the private sector. The cost, conversely, is that the research *within* each organisation was limited in scope and time. In each case we interviewed the headquarters staff responsible for the design and operation of PI systems. In each case, too, we followed this up by selectively interviewing some of those involved at regional and branch level. In each case, finally, we drew on all the available documentation, both published and unpublished. However, we do not purport to offer in this book a detailed, blow by blow study of how each organisation set about inventing and implementing its system of PIs. Nor do we seek to provide any sort of definitive evaluation of the way in which different organisations use performance indicators. The aim is rather to give the reader a sense of how a wide variety of organisations – some of them, like the NHS, much studied while others, like the prison service, rather lower in profile – have set about the difficult task of developing PIs, using the empirical data generated by our research. In doing so, we have sought to identify issues and commonalities across organisations – the common core of conceptual and technical problems involved – as well as the differences between them. It is an exercise which, we hope, will be useful both to those engaged in the practical business of designing and using PIs and to those interested, whether as teachers or students, in the study of how organisations and governments behave.

Our method depended crucially on the help given generously by a large but necessarily anonymous cast in a variety of organisations. In the case of the public sector organisations, the interviews were carried out on lobby terms and we cannot therefore identify the civil servants and others concerned. In the case of the private sector organisations, the interviews were carried out on the understanding that the firms concerned would not be identified or identifiable. Hence our thanks have to be general rather than particular; they are no less sincere for that. We are also grateful to colleagues at the School of Social Sciences at Bath University who contributed their specialist knowledge in particular fields, to Sylvia Hodges and Janet Bryant for organising our work, and to Jane Davies for producing the final text. Finally, we must acknowledge the support of the Economic and Social Research Council who funded our work (grant number E09 250013) and have made this book possible.

Bath, September 1990

POSTSCRIPT TO THE PAPERBACK EDITION

Since we completed the text for the original hardback edition of this book, four years ago, there have been many changes in the political and administrative landscapes. For example, the boundaries between the public and the private sectors continue to shift: the privatisation of water has been completed while the privatisation of the railways is about to begin. But most of the changes that have taken place confirm both the importance of performance indicators as a tool of public management and the continuing relevance of our conceptual framework for thinking about their use and development.

The Thatcherite cultural revolution has indeed outlived its progenitor as far as the machinery of government is concerned. The Next Steps Initiative has continued to accelerate: agencies have proliferated – among them the Social Security delivery system described in Chapter 4. The creation of such agencies was highly dependent on the availability of performance measures, which made hands-off control possible. In turn, the PIs themselves have been modified in order to inform decisions about the allocation of resources. The production of PIs continues to be an expanding, if contentious, industry.

Most contentious of all has been the production of 'populist PIs', i.e. performance indicators which are aimed at the public rather than managers. The league tables for hospitals and schools are the most conspicuous, as well as the most controversial, examples. Their introduction has prompted a public debate about how the performance of such services should be measured, about what indicators should be used and about the interpretation of the information. In this respect, at least, and despite the failure of Parliament to grasp the opportunities offered, we appear to be moving towards realising the hope – expressed in our final paragraph – of rescuing the concept of PIs from the exclusive world of experts and integrating it into the democratic process.

N.C.; R.K.; P.D.   August 1994

1 Revolution or resurrection?

The history of a concept

Just as the start of the French Revolution is conventionally taken to be 14 July 1789, so the start of the Thatcher managerial revolution can be dated with some precision, 17 May 1982. No buildings in Whitehall were stormed, no Bastille fell, and there is unlikely to be dancing in the street on the anniversary of the event in future years. However, on that day the Treasury sent out a note to a variety of government departments (Prime Minister and Minister for the Civil Service 1982) resonant with implications for the inhabitants of the Whitehall village. This called for 'a general and co-ordinated drive to improve financial management in government departments', so launching what came to be known as the Financial Management Initiative (FMI). The principle underlying the FMI was simple and was to be elaborated in countless documents. It was that managers at all levels in government should have 'a clear view of their objectives; and assess, and wherever possible measure, outputs or performance in relation to these objectives'. There were thus three critical, and mutually dependent, components in the new management system. The first was the specification of objectives not only for government policies but for individual units within the government machine. The second was the precise and accurate allocation of costs to particular units of activity and programmes. The third was 'the development of performance indicators and output measures which can be used to assess success in achieving objectives'. The question to be addressed, the Treasury note stressed, is 'where is the money going *and* what are we getting for it?' Accordingly 'systems should be devised to provide answers to both sides of the question wherever and to the extent that it is possible to do so. Relevant information on performance and (where possible) outputs will often be non-financial in character'.

Like the storming of the Bastille, the importance of the Treasury note on 17 May 1982 was largely symbolic in character. It gained its significance from what came before and what came afterwards. It was preceded by a variety of initiatives designed to improve management in Whitehall, notably the efficiency strategy (Metcalfe and Richards 1987). It was sustained by continued Prime Ministerial interest and increasing civil service commitment. But before exploring the birth and development of FMI in greater depth, and examining in particular the development of performance indicators, there is a double paradox to be addressed. This is, first, why a set of rather trite, seemingly self-evident propositions – about the need to link objectives, costs, and outputs systematically – could be seen as being so novel in the context of Whitehall: why, in short, could it be perceived as a challenge to the way in which the British Government machine worked? Second, why did a bundle of ideas that had almost achieved the status of an antique suddenly come into favour, to be seen as the latest managerial wonder drug: given that the FMI was a resurrection rather than a revolution intellectually, why did the concepts embodied in it suddenly achieve a second coming? To provide some answers to these questions, this chapter first explores the intellectual roots of the 1982 initiative, and its emphasis on performance indicators, before returning to look at the specific circumstances that provoked the launch of the FMI and ensured its development over the rest of the decade. For the history of the concepts provides a warning against seeking to interpret the FMI too exclusively in terms of either the characteristics of the Thatcher Administration or of the institutional structures and traditions of Britain.

A CONCEPT AND ITS HISTORY

At the risk of over-simplification, the concepts embodied in the Financial Management Initiative can be seen as a response – one of many – to the growth in the scale and scope of State activity everywhere during the 20th century, and in particular in the period after 1945. Government was becoming not only bigger but also more complex. Its budget expanded in line with its responsibilities. Its organisation changed as, increasingly, it took on service-delivery roles. The cobweb networks of co-ordinating committees grew in intricacy. The result, everywhere, was a perceived lack of control and accountability; the notion of overload was born (King 1975). Ministers no longer felt in control of their departments; Parliament no longer felt that Ministers could be called to account effectively. The lack of transparency of government activities reinforced the sense of paralysed helplessness in the face of size and complexity. In Britain, the result throughout the 1960s was a debate about the machinery of government (see, for example, Thomas 1968 and Crick 1968), ranging from Whitehall to

Westminster and beyond. The decade was, consequently, marked by continuing pressure to adapt existing institutions and to devise new tools in order to make big government more manageable and more efficient.

Nor was this phenomenon exclusive to Britain. It was the United States which produced much of the vocabulary and many of the techniques that shaped a variety of initiatives in this country, and ultimately the FMI. In 1961 the US Department of Defense introduced a planning, programming, budgeting (PPB) system devised and directed by Charles Hitch, a former Rand Corporation analyst, in order to assert central control for the effective use of resources. It was a department marked by its vast budget, its difficulties in dealing with runaway procurement costs, and the ambitious obduracy of the military in seeking as many and as sophisticated weapons as possible (Hitch 1965). Its Secretary, Robert McNamara, had every incentive to seek a better instrument of control and decision-making. Subsequently, in 1965, President Johnson promulgated that PPB systems should be adopted by all civilian agencies of the federal government. PPB, or output budgeting as it became known, had the following objectives:

1 To define the objectives of policies in all major areas of government activity.
2 To organise information about expenditure and use of resources in terms of the specific programmes designed to achieve these objectives.
3 To analyse the output of programmes so as to have some measurement of their effectiveness.
4 To evaluate alternative ways of achieving the same policy objectives, and to achieve these objectives for the least cost.
5 To formulate objectives and programmes over a period of years, and to provide feedback about the appropriateness and effectiveness of the methods chosen.

(Schultze 1968: 19–23)

The PPB system was therefore designed, and seen, as an instrument for planning government activities more rationally, more efficiently, and more effectively. It was, in this respect, very much the product of the era of faith in managerial rationalism (Challis et al. 1988), before the faith was challenged by economic crisis and political disillusion in the 1970s. Indeed it was explicitly argued that the rationality of planning was preferable to – and more equitable than – the rationality of politics. The normative case for adopting a systems approach, as developed in a notable analysis by Schick (1969), deserves exploring at some length since its relevance has not diminished over the decades. Decision-making through 'process politics', Schick argued, inevitably tends to 'favor partisans such as agencies, bureaus and interest groups'. Legitimated by pluralistic theory, the process approach furthermore offers 'a convenient escape from difficult value questions'. Whatever is produced through the process of bargaining, is best: 'once they were sold on the efficiency of interest groups, the pluralists stopped worrying about the ends of government. They were persuaded by a tautological, but nonetheless alluring, proof that the outcomes of the group process are satisfactory'. Moreover, the persuasiveness of the pluralistic model of decision-making depended heavily – as Schick noted already in 1969 – on taking growing economic affluence for granted, so that politics was seen as 'a giant positive sum game in which almost everyone comes out ahead' and on assuming that even disadvantaged groups were able to take part in the bargaining.

In contrast, the systems approach – of which PPB was an off-spring – was designed to produce 'an explicit examination of outcomes'. Unlike the process model, it did not have an in-built bias towards the stronger actors in the political arena. By demonstrating unsatisfactory outcomes, it might furthermore provoke criticism of the political processes which had produced them: Schick indeed argued that the 'systems mood' of the 1960s in the United States reflected the rediscovery of poverty and racial inequalities. PPB can thus, in a sense, be seen as giving visibility to minority interests denied voice in the normal political processes. Moreover, the systems approach involved a shift in the distribution of power in a double sense. Not only is it about the distribution of power within society; it is also about the distribution of power within the government machine. As Schick pointed out:

> In the usual bureaucratic pattern, budgetary power is located at the lower echelons, with successively higher levels having declining power and less involvement. By the time the budget reaches the President, most of the decisions have been made for him in the form of existing programs and incremental bureau claims. Barring unusual exertion, the President's impact is marginal, cutting some requests and adding some items of his own.
>
> (Schick 1969: 143)

The introduction of PPB could thus be seen as a way of strengthening the ability of the President to impose his will: more generally 'systems politics tends to favor the central allocators, especially the chief executive and the budget agency'. Substitute Prime Minister for President, and the implications are clear, particularly for Prime Ministers with a presidential temperament.

By 1969, when Schick was writing, enthusiasm for PPB was on the wane in the United States. It was sharply criticised by the pluralists (for example, Wildavsky 1979). As Schick conceded:

> PPB is an idea whose time has not quite come. It was introduced government wide before the requisite concepts, organisational capability, political conditions, informational resources, and techniques were adequately developed. A decade ago, PPB was beyond reach; a decade or two hence, it, or some updated version, might be one of the conventions of budgeting.
>
> (Schick 1969: 50)

However, he also concluded that a systems approach 'might mean permanent crisis' and 'constant struggle over public ends and means', by giving visibility to outcomes, while process politics was designed to avoid such conflict. Hence systems politics would never replace process politics. It is a conclusion that suggests, if only tentatively, that a systems approach is likely to be adopted only by a government with a high degree of tolerance for conflict.

As so often, just as the United States was beginning to become disillusioned with an idea, it was being imported with enthusiasm into Britain (Klein 1972). The Ministry of Defence decided in 1964 to adopt a system similar to that already introduced by its American counterpart. Subsequently the Treasury decided to experiment with 'output budgeting', as PPB was rechristened. And in 1970 the Department of Education and Science (DES) published a feasibility study of applying output budgeting techniques to its activities (DES 1970). But what was originally intended as a model for other Ministries to follow turned out in practice to be the obituary for the new technique. Although the Department of Health and Social Security produced what it styled a programme budget (Banks 1979), involving the allocation of expenditures to certain broad heads of activity (like services for the elderly), little more was heard about output budgeting. Conceptually and technically, 'output budgeting' had proved difficult to translate into an operational system; in particular, the definition of outputs and the development of indicators of success had turned out to be an elusive task, a point to which we return below. The attempt had also tended to soak up time and scarce expertise in the civil service; the investment costs had turned out to be very high. Above all, the early 1970s saw the birth of a new generation of acronyms: the fashions in managerial radicalism had changed. The 1970 White Paper on *The Reorganisation of Central Government* (Prime Minister 1970) – the managerial manifesto of the Heath Administration, just as the FMI was the managerial manifesto of the Thatcher Administration – still stressed the need 'for explicit statements of the objectives of expenditure in a way that would enable a Minister's plans to be tested against general government strategy'. However, it also launched a new concept: Programme Analysis and Review (PAR). So PAR replaced PPB, only to vanish in turn by the middle of the 1970s (Heclo and Wildavsky 1981) – not before, however, the DES had once again pioneered the new technique and carried out a departmental PAR under the Secretaryship of Margaret Thatcher.

Although the fashions in acronyms changed from decade to decade, there was remarkable stability over time in the concerns (and the interests voicing them) underlying the various attempts to bring new techniques into British Government. They can conveniently be analysed under three headings, although in practice there was considerable overlap between the categories; (1) concern about public expenditure planning, (2) concern about the managerial competence of Whitehall, and (3) concern about accountability. The initial impulse for devising new instruments and techniques of control came from alarm about the incremental but inexorable upward drift in public spending: the result was the Plowden Report (Chancellor of the Exchequer 1961) which gave birth to a new system of public expenditure control and subsequently led to the publication of an annual Public Expenditure White Paper (Klein 1989b). Its emphasis was on devising a system that would allow long-term planning and force a more critical scrutiny of commitments, both new and old, by Parliament and public in the expectation that this would lead to greater restraint in spending. The expectation was not to be realised, even though it was shared by the Treasury. The second strand, what might be called ministerial concerns although they were not exclusive to them by any means, reflected the feeling that the problems of modern government had outrun the capacity of the civil service to cope with them and that structural change was needed: a point already touched on. This was to lead to the appointment in 1966 of the Fulton Committee on the Civil Service (Fulton 1968), and a string of proposals for introducing managerial ideas into Whitehall. Lastly, there was continuing concern in Parliament not only about the control of public expenditure and the competence of government, but also about the lack of accountability that followed from the sheer complexity of the spending process and the lack of accessibility to the managerial process in Whitehall: hence a succession of demands, spanning the decades from the 1960s into the 1980s, calling for a system that would produce both greater efficiency and more transparency.

There were, then, at least three constituencies with an interest in promoting change though not necessarily change of the same kind or at the same pace: the Treasury, Ministers, and Parliament. At times, their interests diverged; the emphasis shifted, at different periods, from expenditure control to managerial worries, from managerial worries to issues of accountability, and back again; on occasions environmental turbulence, notably economic crisis, displaced all three and pushed more immediate issues to the forefront. However, given the underlying continuity, it is worth analysing briefly some of the arguments and proposals of the 1960s, since they were to surface again in the 1980s albeit in a new language. Specifically the Fulton Committee anticipated (ibid.: Ch. 5) much of the logic underlying the 1982 FMI. It argued that efficiency in government, as in all large organisations, required delegation of responsibility; in turn, such delegation required a structure in which units and individuals could be held accountable for the achievement of specified objectives. In a section (para. 150) that could well have been included in the 1982 Treasury note, the Committee argued:

> Accountable management means holding individuals and units responsible for performance measured as objectively as possible. Its achievement depends upon identifying or establishing accountable units within government departments – units where output can be measured as objectively as possible and where individuals can be held personally responsible for their performance
>
> (Fulton 1968: 51)

Here, then, is the emphasis on 'measurable output' – or alternative, non-quantitative criteria for assessing performance – that was to characterise the 1980s initiative. And here, too, was a stress on 'hiving off' government activities to independent boards or bodies, which was yet another concern of the 1980s: suggesting that we are perhaps drawing on a package of linked ideas – a sort of a political ideology of managerial reform in government – forged in the 1960s but destined to resurface in a very different environment twenty years later.

Certainly a remarkable continuity and consensus is evident in a succession of parliamentary reports spanning two decades, originating from a variety of House of Commons Committees and bearing the signatures of a long succession of MPs drawn from all parties. It was driven by the ambition to re-assert, in new circumstances, the traditional parliamentary function of controlling and scrutinising public spending. But the traditional concern was clothed in a new language: so, for example, in 1969 the House of Commons asserted that its role was to ensure that public spending should be 'efficiently planned and managed'. The same report endorsed the notion of 'output budgeting':

> Output budgeting is of great significance to the House of Commons for two reasons. First, by setting out the activities of Departments in the form of costed programmes, it will enable the House to weigh the objectives selected by Departments against possible alternatives. Second, the development of output budgeting will increase the possibilities of assessing Departments' efficiency in setting objectives and their measure of success in realising them.
>
> (Select Committee on Procedure 1969: xii)

The influence of American ideas is clear; the Committee had sent its Clerk to study the PPB system in Washington. And the same theme was taken up in a series of parliamentary reports stretching over the 1970s. Even though the fires of enthusiasm for output budgeting and indicators of success had died down in Whitehall, Westminster insisted on trying to breathe new life into the dying embers. In 1971 the Expenditure Committee called for spending plans to be linked to objectives, and for at least some measures of output (Expenditure Committee 1971 para. 19). The following year, the Committee called for a new information system:

> The idea of a comprehensive set of statistics of outputs over the whole range of public expenditure is an ambitious one. But we believe that it ought to be regarded as a realistic and reasonable aim. Patient work by the civil service and computer techniques have given us, through measurement of expenditure at constant prices, one of the most sophisticated analyses of inputs in the world; we think that the possibilities inherent in the present system will not be fully realised until the analysis of inputs is matched by an analysis of outputs.
>
> (Expenditure Committee 1972: ix)

Implicit in these, and similar, demands from Parliament was a revolution in the concept of accountability for public spending. For centuries, Parliament had fought to establish its right to examine – and in theory to veto – proposals for spending. Now it was fighting for its right to examine what the money had actually bought. The importance of this change is well caught in the following quotation from Alice Rivlin, one of the apostles of the new systems approach in the United States whose influence was to stretch into the 1980s:

> ... stating accountability in terms of inputs – through detailed guidelines and controls on objects of expenditure – spawns red tape

and rigidity without introducing incentives to more outputs. Hence a new approach is in order: state the accountability in terms of outputs, and reward those who produce more efficiently.

(Rivlin 1971: 126–7)

Rivlin's point was made in the context of a discussion of Congressional control over spending. The fact that it echoes discussions of parliamentary control over public expenditure is significant, and this for two reasons. First, it tends to confirm that the interest in devising new techniques, of which performance indicators formed an essential part, was a cross-national response to a shared set of problems. Second, it demonstrates yet again the existence of a set of ideas whose persistence reflected, in part at least, the fact that they were expounded by a permanent intellectual lobby whose influence was growing from the 1960s onwards.

In effect, the advocates of the systems approach argued – as already noted – that the rationality of politics was not enough. It required to be supplemented, if not replaced, by a model of rationality largely drawn from economics. The drive for better budgetary systems, the identification of objectives, and the measurement of outputs coincided with, and to an extent reflected, the rise of the 'econocrats' in government (Self 1975). The intellectual history of the influence of economists and their notions on the techniques of government still waits to be written. But it is evident that it was growing rapidly from the 1960s onwards, on both sides of the Atlantic. Not only were more economists at work in Whitehall: their presence in the offices of Ministers was already being compared to the role of domestic chaplains in the courts of mediaeval monarchs. But their ideas were permeating the training of civil servants, who were being introduced to the language of cost–benefit analysis and similar notions. So in 1967 the Treasury's Centre for Administrative Studies – a precursor of the Civil Service College – published a study of output budgeting (Williams 1967): a study which firmly anchored this concept in the context and traditions of micro-economics. The missionary enterprise was not limited to Whitehall. Significantly, economists were also involved in the production of the various parliamentary committee reports, whether as advisers or as contributors of memoranda of evidence. Moreover, their ideas appealed because they were drawn not only from micro-economics but also from a tradition of applying analytical techniques to public policy problems which goes back to at least the time of Edwin Chadwick (1867), who saw expertise, information, and openness as essential safeguards against the power of what he called 'the baleful money interests': i.e. very much the same ethical justification for applying rational analytical methods to government decisions that was put forward 100 years later for the development of the PPB system in the United States. In a sense, the new techniques could be presented as protection for the ruled against the self-interests of the rulers, Ministers and civil servants alike.

The ambitious claims of the 'econocrats' were, in turn, to produce a backlash. It quickly became apparent that some of the claims made for their techniques had out-run their capacity to deliver the goods. The gap between theory and practice – particularly in the area of cost–benefit analysis – proved to be a yawning one. Similarly, it became evident that measuring the output of government in the one currency with which economists are comfortable, money, was not feasible: the outputs of government stubbornly refused to be reduced to a single dimension or denominator. The point is clearly illustrated by the 1970 feasibility study of output budgeting in the Department of Education and Science, already cited. It endorsed the idea of output budgeting as a way of compelling decision-makers to think more clearly about what they were doing. Specifically, it argued that such a system would force policy makers to direct their attention not at activities but at the impact of those activities on the environment: i.e. on final objectives or outcomes rather than intermediate outputs. For example, the 'effectiveness of the housing programme may best be judged, not by the number of dwellings built, but by the number of households housed (and re-housed)'. But in making this point, the feasibility study identified the real problem: that in most cases it was impossible to measure outcomes: i.e. the impact on society. Nor did the difficulties stop there. First, there was the problem of multiple or contested objectives. Second, if intermediate outputs (such as pupil/teacher ratios) were used instead of final output or outcome measures, it was essential that 'the relationship between intermediate and final outputs should be understood'. Third, there was inevitably a time-lag between activity and impact, particularly in a programme like education where the benefits only become fully apparent over decades.

All these issues are fully explored in the next chapter. What needs noting here is the conclusion drawn by the DES feasibility study. On the one hand, it argued against an exclusive preoccupation with 'quantification' in the assessment of performance. On the other hand, it pointed out that any attempt to measure output would require research and special studies; while indicators of activity could be derived from routinely collected administrative statistics, these were an inadequate tool for measuring performance in the more ambitious sense of the word. In short, the DES report suggested that in 1970 output budgeting was still largely a concept in search of the tools required to make it work: what the economists had produced was a manifesto of future aspirations rather than a set of techniques which could be used in the present.

However, to complete our cast list of those involved in the performance indicators movement, there was another set of actors anxious to demonstrate that they could fill the gap left by the economists: the social science community as a whole. The rise of interest in what came to be known as social indicators mirrors that of the story of output budgeting. It began in the United States in the mid-sixties and came to Britain at the end of the decade. The aim was to complement economic indicators with social indicators: if society was growing richer, was it also getting healthier, safer, happier, and so on? A year after decreeing that PPB should flourish universally, President Johnson directed that the Department of Health, Education and Welfare should develop a set of 'social statistics and indicators' so that 'we can better measure the distance we have come and plan the way ahead'. The resulting report – prepared in the office of Alice Rivlin, then Assistant Secretary in the Department, under the direction of Mancur Olson – had the same touch of radical rationalism that characterised many of the advocates of PPB. The case for social indicators, it argued, was both to give 'social problems more visibility' and, ultimately, to 'make possible a better evaluation of what public programs are accomplishing'. And it concluded:

> The social statistics that we need will almost never be obtained as a by-product of accounting or administrative routine, or as a result of a series of *ad hoc* decisions, however intelligent each of these decisions might be. Only a systematic approach based on the informational requirement of public policy will do.
>
> (US Department of Health, Education and Welfare 1969: 101)

The American movement of ideas found a sympathetic response in Britain. It enlisted the interest of Claus Moser, the then head of the Central Statistical Office, and the result was the annual publication of *Social Trends*, starting in 1970. In 1971 Andrew Shonfield, then chairman of the Social Science Research Council, organised a meeting at Ditchley for British social scientists with an interest in social indicators to meet some of their American counterparts. But the current of academic interest was beginning to run just as the tide of political support for the development of new tools of government was on the turn. In the volume that emerged from the Ditchley conference there was what turned out to be a prophetic last chapter by Richard Rose on the market for policy indicators. This concluded that

> ... new social indicators might most readily gain acceptance and long-range importance in so far as they initially supported existing policies and implied no cost of action. It is much easier to get people to accept the outside evaluation implicit in social indicators if the result is favourable.
>
> (Rose 1972: 140)

With Britain about to enter a period of economic turbulence, the market disappeared. What was left, however, was a stock of ideas and a potential constituency for a re-birth of interest in a new environment in the 1980s.

THE SECOND COMING

By the middle of the 1970s commitment to, and enthusiasm about, the new managerialism had waned; government was preoccupied with more urgent matters. Public expenditure appeared to be out of control (Wright 1977); a crisis which, in turn, seemed to undermine many of the assumptions of the reformers. Perversely, a public expenditure control system devised to bring about more rationality in the allocation and use of resources had the consequence of encouraging irrational spending decisions: the presentation of expenditure decisions in constant price figures, designed to facilitate long-term planning, had the effect of diverting the attention of Ministers from the cash costs of their commitments (Pliatzky 1982). So PPB, PAR, and all the rest were forgotten while the Treasury concentrated on bringing spending under control by introducing a system of cash limits. The search for solvency displaced the search for efficiency; the emphasis on economy, or cutting costs, took precedence over concern with effectiveness. So, for example, the Government's statistical services were cut, thereby reducing its capacity to generate the kind of information subsequently needed for PIs. The manifesto of the incoming 1979 Thatcher Administration (Conservative Central Office 1979) emphasised the need to cut public spending rather than managerial reform in Whitehall. It promised that 'the reduction of waste, bureaucracy and over-government will yield substantial savings'. And indeed among the first initiatives taken by the new Prime Minister was the creation of an Efficiency Unit – headed by Sir Derek (subsequently Lord) Rayner, joint managing director of Marks and Spencer – designed to promote value for money throughout Whitehall and beyond. It was an initiative which had three main characteristics (Metcalfe and Richards 1987). First, the Efficiency Unit was very much the Prime Minister's own creature: it was housed in the Prime Minister's office and reported directly to her. Second, it carried out a series of quick, small-scale scrutinies of specific expenditure programmes. Third, and perhaps most important from the perspective of this analysis, its style and strategy reflected Rayner's conviction that it was more important to change the managerial culture in Whitehall than to introduce changes in the managerial machinery. Unlike the innovations of the 1960s and early 1970s, the efficiency enterprise was therefore not led by techniques or experts. It was designed to harness the experience and enthusiasm of civil servants to the search for greater efficiency rather than to bring about a revolution in the technology of public administration or to introduce the skills of economists into Whitehall. Similarly, while the Efficiency Unit provided a model for the search for greater efficiency in government, it did not institutionalise it: the Unit owed (and owes) its effectiveness precisely to the fact that it is the Prime Minister's personal instrument and remains outside the normal routines of the civil service – that it makes occasional raids into specific areas rather than carrying out a comprehensive or systematic review of all activities.

The 1982 Financial Management Initiative, in contrast, represented a move to institutionalise the search for efficiency and to generalise the attempts to change the managerial culture of Whitehall. That the move should have taken the form of adopting concepts and techniques developed in the era of Harold Wilson and Ted Heath – that a government dedicated to the ideology of the market should have drawn on the tradition of rational, corporate planning – may, at first sight, appear surprising. In fact, the reasons are plain. If the original systems approach was developed in the 1960s in response to dawning worries about growing public expenditure, by the 1980s those worries had become overriding, dominating concerns for all governments but particularly so for the Thatcher Administration. Any machinery of control and analysis which put the emphasis on the *outputs* of government – instead of defining all improvements in terms of *inputs* – was therefore calculated to appeal in the circumstances of the 1980s. Given, too, that the language of the FMI was also the vocabulary of business management, it is not surprising that the Thatcher Government learnt to use it despite its earlier associations.

There were other factors at work too. Specifically, there was the desire of some Ministers to get a grip over their own departments: to ensure that the civil servants, for whose activities they were accountable to Parliament, were actually accountable to them. It was this which led

Michael Heseltine to develop what in some respects was a precursor of the FMI, the Management Information System for Ministers (MINIS) at the Department of the Environment. This sought to identify centres of activities, allocate costs to them, and link them to objectives. However, as Heseltine records:

> On one memorable occasion, I was asked by the Prime Minister to give my colleagues an account of how MINIS was helping the DOE to put its house in order. My fellow Cabinet ministers sat in rows while I explained my brainchild, each with his sceptical permanent secretary behind him muttering objections, or so I suspected. Any politician knows when he is losing his audience's attention, and I knew well enough. When I had done, there were few takers and absolutely no enthusiasts.
>
> (Heseltine 1987: 22)

But the pressures were building up. In particular, there was continuing pressure from Parliamentary Committees, making many of the same points (and indeed using some of the same specialist advisers) that had provided the themes of their reports in the 1970s and earlier. Some of those reports were specific to particular Ministries, and helped to shape departmental responses: Chapter 4 provides an example of this in the case of the Department of Health and Social Security. Above all, there was the report of the Treasury and Civil Service Committee (1982) that provoked the Government to announce the launching of the FMI in its response to the parliamentary criticism.

The arguments of the Treasury and Civil Service Committee are worth setting out in some detail because they bring out the centrality of performance measures or indicators in the kind of management system advocated in its report and, to a large extent, embodied in the FMI concept. The conclusion of the Committee (para. 48) was brutally wounding for an Administration that prided itself on its value for money zeal:

> There is no clear orientation towards the achievement of effectiveness and efficiency at the higher levels of the Civil Service or in government generally. While the broad intentions of policy are often clear enough there are too few attempts to set operational objectives and realistic targets against which to measure the outturn. Measures of output are inadequate. Consequently there are no systematic means of guiding and correcting the use of resources.
>
> (Treasury and Civil Service Committee 1982: xxiv)

There was 'commendable concern with economy in the use of resources', the Committee conceded. But this should not be confused with either effectiveness or efficiency. It pointed out that the measures of output used by departments – such as the number of payments made or patients treated – 'say little about the effectiveness of a programme and they are of small value for assessing the progress being made towards the real objectives'. Similarly, cuts in civil service numbers or savings made as the result of Rayner scrutinies did not necessarily mean greater efficiency, if the result meant a reduction in outputs or led to 'a programme being administered less equitably than before'. Furthermore, in its failure to set explicit objectives, and devise means of measuring progress towards their achievement, government compared badly with business organisations. 'Ministers should not be able to escape accountability by not declaring objectives and targets', the Committee concluded, 'They account continuously to Parliament for the resources used, and they should account for the results achieved in relation to objectives and targets'. And within the government machine, the Committee argued, echoing the recommendations of the Fulton Report, 'There should be greater devolution of management but strengthened central review of the effectiveness and efficiency with which management operates'.

There were, then, a number of different arguments pointing in the same direction – the need to develop measures of performances. On the one hand, there were the managerial arguments. There could be no way of assessing progress in achieving greater efficiency and effectiveness without such measures. Similarly, the decentralisation of government activities inevitably meant centralising knowledge about what they were doing (Perrow 1977). On the other hand, there were the political arguments. If the constitutional fiction of ministerial accountability to Parliament was to be made a reality, then it was essential to devise currencies of evaluation that would allow MPs to scrutinise the departmental record. Similarly, Ministers themselves had to develop instruments which would allow them to get a grip on their own activities. Lastly, there was an element hitherto not touched on: accountability to the public. In 1981 the Department of the Environment issued a Code of Practice (DoE 1981) exhorting local authorities to include in their annual reports 'a short list of performance statistics'. Such indicators, the Code of Practice suggested, might include comparisons with other authorities, trends over time and between plans and achievements. The indicators might 'measure one or more of the various aspects of performance, including the cost, scale and quality of service, the demand for the service, the degree of client satisfaction, relative efficiency and so on'. No doubt one intention in this was to bring pressure on local authorities to reduce the rate of increase in spending: to mobilise public opinion against extravagance. However, the initiative demonstrated that there could be a populist, as well as a managerial, dimension to the case for producing performance indicators. And although the main impulse behind the FMI may have been the traditional concern about getting value for money out of public expenditure, it is clear that the resulting emphasis in measuring performance had wider implications for the style of government.

THE PERFORMANCE OF PIs: POST-1982

Following the Financial Management Initiative, performance indicators did indeed multiply. In 1985 the annual Public Expenditure White Paper contained 500 output and performance measures. In the two succeeding years, the figures rose first to 1200 and then to 1800. And by the time that the 1988 White Paper was published, the PI explosion had been such that no one was counting any more (Carter 1988). There could be no better illustration of the zeal that departments bring to a task once it has been promulgated by the Treasury with the backing of the Prime Minister. The problems and strategies of a variety of departments are examined in subsequent chapters. Here we are only concerned with the broad picture. And this would suggest that Whitehall proved more skilful in presenting existing statistics and information in the guise of PIs rather than successful in developing new measures designed to meet the requirements of the FMI. The explosion of PIs in the White Paper represented a presentational triumph rather than marking a managerial revolution: evidence of the skill of civil servants in conforming with the latest swing in Whitehall fashions, as dictated by the Treasury, rather than of any fundamental shift in bureaucratic attitudes.

Some examples, taken from the 1990 Public Expenditure White Paper (HM Treasury 1990: Cmnd. 1001, 1008), make the point. They are taken from departments not subsequently examined in this study. The Ministry of Defence gives the following examples of performance indicators being used in the Department: costs per vehicle mile, cost per unit of equipment used, plant utilisation, and availability. The Department of the Environment rather more ambitiously relates outputs to targets: for instance, the number of jobs created or preserved in inner area programmes or the number of visitors to royal parks. In short, departments tended to re-christen existing statistics of activity or costing information as performance indicators or measures of output. Moreover, departments appear to be more enthusiastic about introducing PIs designed to assess the performance of their agencies than about measuring their own (Flynn *et al.* 1988). In short, while the White Paper PIs provide a plethora of statistics about activity and a lot of information about costings, there is relatively little that allows conclusions to be drawn about efficiency and effectiveness in government.

However, it would be a mistake to conclude from this that, as far as PIs are concerned, the FMI revolution has turned out to be cosmetic rather than cultural: that Whitehall has only learnt to apply a new label to existing statistics, and that nothing has changed. The very fact of re-labelling may, in itself, be of significance: a signal that a department is using statistics of activity, rather than merely collecting them as a matter of tradition and routine. Moreover, any conclusions drawn from the Public Expenditure White Papers needed to be qualified by other evidence. What they do not reveal is the sustained drive by the Treasury to make the language of self-evaluation, and with it the vocabulary of output and performance measurement, part of the normal trading relationship between it and other government departments. It is a strategy which starts at the top: in making a case for extra money, for new programmes or initiatives, Cabinet Ministers have to state their objectives and the criteria to be used in assessing progress towards their achievement. And there has been continuing pressure on departments to produce case studies of self-evaluation exercises (HM Treasury 1986a, 1987) from the Treasury Unit responsible for the missionary work of promoting performance measurement.

The case studies suggest some tentative conclusions. The first is that the development of performance indicators appears to have been fastest, because least problematic, in relatively simple sub-units of government with clearly defined functions. These account for a majority of the published case studies, and include the Driver and Vehicle Licensing Centre, the Naval Aircraft Repair Organisation, the Vehicle Inspectorate, and the Chessington Computer Centre. In some instances, the use of PIs seems to be ancient history: thus Her Majesty's Stationery Office records that 'for over a decade HMSO has been measuring its performance and publishing performance indicators'. Second, and conversely, the problems of measuring performance increase with the complexity of government activities: when it comes to large programmes, perhaps with multiple or ill-defined objectives, the task becomes much more formidable. Thus a Treasury review of departmental budgetary processes noted:

> The absence of a coherent methodology for the aggregation of output and performance indicators for higher levels of management. Indeed the need for a hierarchy of information for successive layers of management is not always recognised. Because lower level indicators,

where they exist, are not properly integrated into top management systems, senior officials do not have available all the necessary information for decision making.

(HM Treasury 1986b: 29)

While recognising the problems of devising adequate performance measures, and the dangers of sending the wrong signals, the Treasury report continued to urge departments to tackle this complex task 'pragmatically': it concluded that 'gradual progress towards the "best" should not delay the use of the "good"'.

Much the same picture, of departments chipping away at recalcitrant marble, emerged from a report by the National Audit Office (NAO 1986) and the follow-up inquiry by the Public Accounts Committee (PAC 1987) into the implementation of the Financial Management Initiative. The Comptroller and Auditor General summed up the evidence as follows:

There are inherent difficulties in assessing the effectiveness of programme expenditure though the central departments and the spending departments drew attention to the difficulties created by imprecise, broad, policy objectives; the multiple objectives of programmes; and the difficulty of distinguishing the effects of programmes from other factors. In many cases it had so far proved possible to assess the effect of programmes only in terms of intermediate rather than final outputs.

(National Audit Office 1986: 8)

The same point was taken up by the Public Accounts Committee which, in line with its parliamentary predecessors over the decades, continued to push for the 'setting of clear and preferably quantified objectives' in order 'to provide yardsticks against which to measure performance'. And reinforcing the sense that the debate about managerial techniques and structures in Whitehall is one where successive generations of actors have simply read out the scripts bequeathed to them by their predecessors, the civil servants giving evidence to the Committee produced arguments familiar since the 1960s. As the Head of the Treasury/Cabinet Office Joint Management Unit put it, 'The reason why departments are not further ahead than they are is not in any sense a lack of will, it is because the subjects are intrinsically very difficult. Government activity is very hard to measure' (Public Accounts Committee 1987: 17).

In succeeding chapters we analyse just how hard government activity is to measure and the extent to which the public sector is indeed unique in this respect. However, the history of the last two decades also underlines that the problems are more than conceptual. The problems of implementing the FMI stem not just from the formidable practical difficulties involved but also from the fact that it is intended to challenge the way in which the public sector has gone about its business for a century or more. In the words of Sir Peter Middleton, the Treasury's Permanent Secretary, giving evidence to the Public Accounts Committee: 'this is a hearts and minds exercise'. But while some minds have been converted, as the evidence reviewed above suggests, it is less clear as yet whether Whitehall hearts are beating to the new tune. Thus the 1987 PAC report was concerned that 'scepticism and mistrust of FMI seems to be widespread among middle and lower management grades'. And the following year, the Efficiency Unit's review of management changes in Whitehall since 1979, entitled *The Next Steps* (Jenkins *et al.* 1988) was more critical still. It noted that 'the changes of the last seven years have been important in beginning to shift the focus of attention away from process towards results'. But it concluded that senior management in Whitehall continued to be dominated by those with skills in policy formulation rather than management, that too little attention was being paid to the results to be achieved, and that the nature of the public expenditure negotiations between the Treasury and the departments was such that the latter felt that 'it is inputs which still really matter'. From this followed a radical set of recommendations, including the massive decentralisation of activities from Whitehall and the creation of organisational units where managers have more freedom and more incentives to perform well. Such a decentralisation of activity would require, in turn, budgetary systems that allowed the efficiency and effectiveness of agencies to be monitored, as the Treasury and Civil Service Committee (1988) stressed in its follow-up to the Efficiency Unit's Report. The Committee urged the Government to ensure that the difficulties in producing measures of efficiency are overcome, 'so that the pace of reform is not necessarily slowed'.

The echoes of the Fulton Report, published twenty years earlier, are clear; history would appear to have come full circle. Just as the FMI represented the resurrection of ideas first put forward two decades earlier, so its subsequent history appears to be mirroring the previous experience: organisational suspicion and inertia, leading to a faltering and stuttering process of implementation. However, it would be a mistake to conclude from this that Managerial Revolutions are inevitably bound to end up as Whitehall Restorations: that the ***ancien régime*** is, in fact, indestructible. The evidence reviewed in this chapter can, more plausibly, be interpreted as demonstrating the persistence and tenacity of the forces with an interest in the promotion of change as well as the difficulties (conceptual as well as organisational) in carrying it out The analysis in subsequent chapters of the experience and strategies of various organisations in developing and using performance indicators and output measures is therefore designed not only to illuminate the process so far but also to provide an input for what is certain to be a continuing process of adaptation, innovation, and evolution. As the FMI yields to *The Next Steps*, as the manifesto of the Whitehall radicals, so there will be a new context and perhaps also a new vocabulary. But this seems likely, to anticipate the conclusion of our last chapter, to reinforce rather than diminish interest in the measurement of performance.

2 Models, measures, and muddles

Organisational and conceptual dimensions of performance indicators

Clearly, the long-running saga of managerial reform in government is still able to sustain audience interest; even if, just like all good soap operas, the same plots (and characters) seem to reappear at regular intervals. It is time now to take a closer look at some of the underlying themes that make up the plot; to analyse the conceptual significance of the story. If the first chapter is regarded as a history of the movement of managerial reform – an account of events – then this chapter offers a review of the arguments spawned by these developments. But it is not simply a history of ideas. It also sets out our approach to the comparative study of performance measurement in public and private organisations. The tone is deliberately speculative: our approach does not provide all the answers, rather it provides a helpful way into a more informed discussion about complex issues that have perplexed public managers for more than two decades.

It is apparent from the history of the movement that organisations have developed systems of performance indicators at varying speeds. This suggests that differences between them and between the modes of service delivery will profoundly influence the form, appropriateness, and use of performance indicators. These differences may result from factors that are specific to particular organisational types – whether, for example, there is one objective or multiple, conflicting, objectives – or from certain generic problems of performance assessment, such as the difficulty in measuring the quality of service delivery. Consequently, our contention is that many of the problems of performance assessment transcend the public/private distinction and reflect characteristics which cut across this particular divide. In the first part of this chapter, we set out the organisational dimensions that we found most useful in helping to analyse differences in the design and use of PIs across our set of case studies.

As the previous chapter showed, the designers of performance indicators in the public sector (and, we would contend, the private sector) have had to grapple with some complex concepts: inputs and outputs, efficiency and effectiveness, the problems of comparing like with like; the list goes on. The conceptual and semantic confusion surrounding these ideas has, in turn, generated a literature, with roots in several disciplines, that has multiplied almost as rapidly as the performance indicators themselves. Apart from economics – to which we can turn for help in understanding basic concepts like efficiency – the broad net of interest captures researchers in the overlapping disciplines of management, accountancy, public administration, social policy, and political science. This breadth of interest brings with it a wide variety of concerns: for example, the largely theoretical output of economists is balanced by the more practical output of accountants such as the Chartered Institute of Public Finance and Accountancy (CIPFA 1984) and the Audit Commission (1986). The quality of work inevitably varies; for example, from the analytical rigour of Levitt and Joyce (1987) and the perceptive observations of Pollitt (1986 *inter alia*), to the derivative description of Jowett and Rothwell (1988). We cannot hope to provide a comprehensive review of the entire literature (nor, we are sure, would the reader wish us to inflict such a burden on her or him). Instead, in the second section of this chapter, we seek to identify the main concepts and issues that characterise the debate and to disentangle those themes and questions that we have found central to an understanding of performance assessment and for setting our own research agenda. Lastly, in the third section, where we consider issues and problems arising from the use of PIs, in order to distinguish the main uses of PIs within organisations, we construct a conceptual scheme for categorising PIs. In all this, by drawing out how *others* look at PIs, the second half of this chapter is essentially seeking to clarify how *we* look at PIs.

At this point, it is necessary to re-emphasise the parameters of our research enterprise. Our concern was not with the performance assessment of organisations like the NHS or of Supermarket as total entities, but with the assessment of performance *within* such organisations; hence all our case studies (with the exception of the British Airports Authority) were picked because they involved the control of a large number of sub-agencies or branches – whether health authorities, social security offices, or supermarkets. To explain variations in the design and use of PIs between these organisations, we must start by setting out the main organisational characteristics that appear to influence the development of PIs.

ORGANISATIONAL CHARACTERISTICS

The literature on comparative organisational analysis is notorious for being a conceptual minefield; note, for example, the critical debate surrounding the Aston programme of studies (Pugh and Hickson 1976; Aldrich 1972; Clegg and Dunkerley 1980 *inter alia*), or the complexity of the bureaumetric approach to public sector comparative analysis (Hood and Dunsire 1981; Dunleavy 1989). So, alert to danger, we have attempted no more than to identify selectively some of the key dimensions along which organisations differ which we regard as relevant to the shaping of performance indicators. These dimensions are intended to form a set of benchmarks for analysing variation in the problems of performance measurement. We are not presenting yet another typology that seeks to explain differences in performance or in structure between organisations. Indeed, as our primary concern is with the control of performance *within* organisations this rather simplifies our task, allowing us to be deliberately selective in picking out those characteristics which seem particularly relevant to the control of internal performance.

The obvious place to start our discussion is with the public/private distinction, i.e. the ownership structure of an organisation, if only because of the widely held view that there is so little common ground in performance measurement between the two sectors that the issue is not worthy of comparative exploration. We stress it here not only because it is conventionally held to be the most significant difference but because, when interviewing civil servants engaged in implementing the FMI, we found a near-unanimity that the assessment of performance in the private sector was different (and unquestionably easier). Two broad explanations are commonly used to explain this difference in public/ private performance measurement. The first assumes that because private firms possess the famous bottom line – profit – then performance measurement is a straightforward, incontestable technical procedure; the second focuses on the particular social and political pressures operating on public sector organisations. It seems appropriate therefore to start with these explanations and to use our exploration of them to draw out a number of dimensions that might account for variations in performance assessment between organisations: these are ownership, trading status, competition, accountability, heterogeneity, complexity, and uncertainty (see Table 2.1, p. 34).

To start with, the civil servants interviewed believed it was self-evident that people's performance could be measured by how much profit they made. Performance assessment in this situation, it is assumed, becomes a virtually mechanical churning out of appropriate figures in contrast to the public sector where there is no 'bottom line' and where there may be multiple, conflicting objectives. However, further examination of this view suggests that it is a difficult position to sustain. In short, it is of great importance to appreciate the limitations of profit as a PI of performance of either the people within the organisation or of the organisation itself.

Even at the level of the firm in the market sector, the common belief that profit is a satisfactory PI presents a misleading picture. The accounts raise questions but do not answer them (Vickers 1965). To imagine that profit figures are a mechanical product is to ignore the fact that accountancy is one of the creative arts; often more art than science (Hopwood 1984). This is well illustrated during takeover battles when accountants are apt to manipulate the figures in order to paint a rosy picture of a company. To assess the meaning of profits (or of alternative key indicators such as market share or return on capital) involves forming a judgement on the performance not just of the firm in question but of its competitors, as well as strategic judgements on the long-term effects of current pricing and investment decisions. In short, the 'bottom line' turns out, on closer inspection, to be a Plasticine concept, both malleable and movable across time.

The 'bottom line' becomes even less useful for assessing performance *within* many for-profit organisations. As a manager in Supermarket, one of the private sector organisations examined in Chapter 5, observed:

> We need to distinguish long-term and short-term outcome implications. We are concerned with long-term outcomes, i.e. in our case, long-term profit, but this is not the same as the short-term outcome. In the short-term you can raise profit by cutting service levels, in the long-term this is counterproductive. This, I believe, is why the private sector cannot rely just on the PI of profit. We need other measures of immediate output and outcome which we can review alongside short-term profit in order to assess likely performance against the long-term outcome objective, i.e. long-term profit.

However, the assessment of short- and long-term profits is complicated in those service industries like banks or building societies where it is particularly difficult to construct a simple profit-and-loss account for individual branches. This makes it very hard for the centre to control subordinate branches or agencies; another reason for developing non-profit PIs. All this suggests, as we shall see in Chapter 5, that private sector organisations attribute considerable importance to non-profit PIs because profit alone is an inadequate measure of performance.

If we turn now to *ownership*; implicit in this perspective is the assumption that every public sector organisation operates under common constraints that set it apart from the private sector. Thus public sector organisations pursue political and social goals rather than simple commercial objectives; further, many public sector organisations do not even trade in the market which, arguably, makes the measurement of performance more complex than in the private sector. But where, in practice, should the line be drawn between public and private ownership, given that there are a wide variety of organisational forms spanning this divide? For within the public sector there are, notably, central and local government departments, agencies, trading funds, and public corporations; within the private sector there are sole traders, partnerships, co-operatives, private and public limited companies; lastly, there is a curious mix of hybrid organisations such as jointly owned enterprises where the government retains a share in ownership. Clearly it is absurd to lump organisations together under the simple labels of either 'public' or 'private'; it is surely better to dispense with the public/private dichotomy and to regard ownership as a continuum ranging from pure government department to the individual entrepreneur (Dunsire *et al.* 1988; Perry and Kraemer 1983). It then becomes interesting to see whether the location of an organisation on the continuum is linked to its approach to performance assessment.

It may, alternatively, be more useful to distinguish organisations according to their *trading status*, i.e. whether they are located in the tradable or non-tradable sectors of the economy. This distinction would place those few remaining public enterprises like British Rail and the Post Office in the same category as private corporations. Moreover, even though nationalised industries are constrained by government policies – from the imposition of cash limits on investments to the pursuit of social objectives such as the operation of loss-making rural railway lines – they do have a wide range of financial indicators of performance not available to non-trading organisations like the police or the NHS. And trading operations like Her Majesty's Stationery Office, recently given agency status, have long employed PIs. But we are primarily concerned with non-profit PIs and the control of the performance of individual branches; why might British Rail differ, if it does, from, say, the police in the design and use of its PI system? Given the availability of financial PIs we might expect British Rail to play down the importance of non-financial PIs.

Perhaps the degree of *competition* – the number of organisations providing similar products or services and their share of the market – is a better dimension? This is a particularly significant dimension given that the Thatcher Administration tried to encourage greater competition in the public sector. The problem is that competition could, in theory, lead to a whole variety of PI strategies: from concentrating on those which measure productive efficiency to those which measure the effectiveness of the service provided to customers. In a similar vein, a monopoly (of which there are many amongst our case studies) may decide that it can ignore non-profit PIs because it faces no market threat, or alternatively it may regard non-profit PIs as a means of assessing the standard of its performance. Clearly competitiveness could be a crucial explanatory factor but the nature of the relationship needs to be explored further.

The competitiveness dimension, like trading status, transcends the public/private divide and, in each category, the degree of protected monopoly or competition may vary. So, for example, although British Rail is a public sector monopoly, it has to compete in the broader transport industry against private road and air transport. On the other hand, companies in the for-profit sector differ sharply in the amount of competition they face: there are many organisations in the private sector that, like British Telecom and BAA – the former British Airports Authority – are virtual monopolies, or, like the four largest clearing banks, have long maintained an oligopolistic domination of their product market. Returning to the earlier example, on this competitive dimension there is clearly an opposing argument for expecting British Rail to attribute considerable importance to non-financial PIs in order to prove to consumers (and itself) that it is able to compete with private cars, coaches, and air travel. Public sector organisations are also involved in another market – the competition for shares of the public purse. One might speculate that the pressure to secure government finance will act as a spur to develop PIs that can be used to support a case for extra resources.

A further dimension concerns the extent to which an organisation is politically *accountable*. Most obviously this takes the form of the various statutory requirements to account for performance which have in recent years obliged most public sector organisations to design at least some PIs. The history of these central government reforms was outlined in the previous chapter, but two further initiatives should be mentioned in this context. First, the formation of the Audit Commission in 1983 laid the foundations for a PI manufacturing industry in local government; the Commission exhorted local authorities to develop PIs as a means of improving economy, efficiency, and effectiveness (Audit Commission 1986). Second, the White Paper on Nationalised Industries (HM Treasury 1978) called for the production and publication of key PIs including, where relevant, standard of service PIs. Nor are these political pressures limited to the public sector. Many of the recently privatised companies are still required to produce standard of service PIs: for example, British Telecom has to report to the Office of Tele-communications (Oftel) and the water industry is now monitored by a number of organisations, including the National Rivers Authority.

Another aspect of accountability may be the extent to which a service is in the public eye and subject to media attention. One might expect that an organisation which is subject to the close scrutiny of consumers with few opportunities to exit and many incentives to exercise voice (such as British Rail) will be compelled to develop PIs against which its performance can be publicly judged. But does this follow? If this is the case, it might be that PIs that are developed primarily for 'outward show' will be different from those which are designed for internal managerial purposes. Again, this is a question that needs to be explored further.

The dimensions discussed so far relate to external political and economic factors arising from the structure of ownership and the nature of the market in which an organisation operates. We now consider a number of organisational dimensions related to the problem of controlling the performance of subordinate branches or agencies which do not fully 'own' their performance. That is, in important respects the performance of an organisation will depend on central decisions and the co-ordination of different streams of activity, as well as their local execution. This would suggest, when making comparisons, the need to look at the distribution of performance ownership as a relevant organisational characteristic, i.e. the extent of discretionary decision-making at different levels in the organisation and the extent of the potential impact of such decisions. In short, who can be held responsible for which dimension or element of performance? The issue of perform-ance ownership applies to both the private and the public sector: whether it be the profitability of individual branches or, as we saw in Chapter 1 for example, the concern of the Fulton Committee with accountable management.

The notion of performance ownership, in turn, raises two further questions. The first is the degree to which performance ownership is constrained by the interdependence of different units, services, or activities within an organisation: if the ability of a unit manager to deliver a good service is constrained by or dependent upon what others do, how far does the individual manager own his or her performance? As we shall see in Chapter 4, the NHS is characterised by a particularly complex set of working relationships, so that the throughput of patients in a hospital may be dependent *inter alia* on radiologists, anaesthetists, surgeons, nurses, and the social workers responsible for finding a place for the discharged patient to go.

The second characteristic concerns the extent to which performance is affected by environmental factors beyond the control of the organisations concerned. For example, the performance of school-children is largely dependent on factors beyond the ambit of the classroom. A league table reporting the exam results of local education authorities will be worthless unless it takes into account the starting place of performance, such as middle-class background or social disadvantage of children (as in Gray and Jesson 1987). Similarly, environmental factors impinge on crime levels. As the Audit Commission (1986) points out, 'How much is vandalism and crime actually reduced by attendance at leisure centres, and how much by the crime prevention and detection activities of the police, or the teaching of social responsibility in schools?' (8).

In drawing together these and other relevant organisational characteristics, we adapted a scheme developed in previous work (Day and Klein 1987), taking from it three dimensions for the assessment of performance which incorporate the above characteristics: hetero-geneity, complexity, and uncertainty.

The first is the degree of *heterogeneity* within any given organisation: by this we mean the number of different products or services provided. The assumption here is that assessing the performance of a single-product organisation is less difficult than assessing that of a multi-product organisation, where there may well be trade-offs between different objectives. Thus, we might expect it to be easier to measure the performance of Social Security branches, where there is arguably just one product – money – than to measure the performance of a hospital where there may be a broad mix of sometimes competing products.

Second, organisations may vary in the degree of *complexity*: by this we mean the extent to which an organisation has to mobilise a number of different skills in order to deliver its services or produce its goods. Complexity may be related to the variety of products delivered by a service but there may also be large variations in the extent to which the co-operation of different skills is required in a single product service. Contrast, for example, the limited number of skills required to provide social security benefits against the many involved in running a surgical unit. The assumption here is that the greater the complexity, the greater also is the scope for interdependence. The greater the interdependence, the more difficult it is to assign the ownership of performance to individual actors or agencies within the organisation. Who exactly was responsible for which bit of performance? It is worth stressing that complexity is separate and distinct from heterogeneity; the police, as we shall see, are low on complexity despite providing a quite heterogeneous set of services.

Third, organisations may vary in the degree of *uncertainty* about the relationship between means and ends; that is, the causal relationship between the input of resources and the achievement of stated objectives. In many organisations, objectives are by no means self-evident. Cyert and March (1963) long ago pointed out that organisations are rarely oriented towards the achievement of any specific goal. Indeed, objectives are often absent, or ambiguous, or phrased in a very general way so as to be not 'operational'. More likely, there will be multiple objectives that are often in conflict. As we shall see, the police carry out several functions, including crime prevention, traffic duties, community relations, and maintaining law and order. The objectives of these activities are not necessarily compatible: a drugs raid in a sensitive inner city area may prevent crime but at the cost of damaging community relations and possibly provoking a breakdown in law and order.

Even if objectives are clear and precise, it is also frequently difficult to establish the relationship between the activities of a service and its impact, and the extent to which performance depends on external actors. If a police force is charged with reducing local crime but is uncertain whether the number of 'bobbies on the beat', the density of neighbourhood watch schemes, or the local level of unemployment will have the greatest impact on crime levels (quite apart from the afore-mentioned environmental factors), then it is difficult to construct a useful PI of police performance. Or, if the objective of the NHS is to improve the health of the nation, is this objective best achieved by the provision of a good health service, or by improving housing and diets? In short, does the service actually 'own' the product for which its performance is being assessed?

We have distinguished seven organisational dimensions which may explain variations in the way services assess their performance. The differences between the organisations studied in this book with respect to these seven dimensions are set out schematically in Table 2.1 and are elaborated in the subsequent chapters. These classifications are obviously rough and ready; they are designed to provide no more than a framework for the study and also to indicate analytical threads that can be followed through and explored when dealing with individual organisations.

In addition, it is useful to bear in mind two more dimensions: the structure of *authority* which refers to the institutional relationship between the centre and periphery, and the *autonomy* of the actors within

Table 2.1 Organisational dimensions

	Owner-ship	Trading/Non-trading	Compet-ition*	Account-ability(1)	Heterogeneity	Complexity	Uncertainty
Police	public	NT	low	yes	med	low	high
Courts	public	NT	low	yes	low	med/high	low
Prisons	public	NT	low	yes	med/low	low	low
Social Security	public	NT	low	yes	low	low	low
NHS	public	NT	low	yes	high	high	high
Supermarket	private	T	high	no	med	med/low	low
High Street Retailer	private	T	high	no	med	med/low	low
Bank	private	T	med→high	no	low	low	low
Building Societies	private	T	med→high	no	low	low	low
Jupiter (TVhire)	private	T	high	no	low	low	low
British Rail	public	T	med	yes	low	low	med
Water (2)	public	T	low	yes	med/low	med	low
BAA	private	T	low	no	low	low	low

* The arrows indicate where an organisation is in the process of change
(1) This refers to formal, public accountability, not actual accountability
(2) This refers to the pre-privatisation water industry

an organisation (Carter 1989). First, organisations vary in the extent to which their institutional structure allows the centre to exercise direct control over the periphery – the local branch or agency. It may be significant that several public sector organisations are characterised by complex lines of responsibility and accountability: illustrated by the arm's length relationship between the Department of Education and local education authorities. The authority structure may provide an incentive to develop PIs, influence the form they take, and have an important impact on their effectiveness.

Second, organisations vary in the degree of autonomy enjoyed by actors within them. In particular, to what extent are administrators prevented from measuring the performance of occupational groups because the distribution of organisational power may concede considerable autonomy to the professional? Central to the notion of professionalism is the assertion that what defines a professional is precisely the fact that he or she is only accountable to his or her peers. It is the professional body that sets the objectives and rules that govern the performance of the individual and it is the profession that defines what is satisfactory performance. Critical to the ability of the government to exercise control over service delivery is the independence of professional accountability from the processes of managerial and political accountability. This independence, combined with the professional claim that their expertise is inevitably incomprehensible to the outsider, makes it difficult for management to impose PIs on professional service deliverers. But autonomy is not the exclusive possession of professionals, and trade union power may on occasion be an adequate substitute for professional status. All aspects of the organisation and control of the work process play a part in the definition of outputs and the apportioning of organisational power. The greater the standardisation of work tasks, the more effectively the centre can measure and control performance; conversely, where the standardisation of work is minimal then the individual worker or group of workers may exercise considerable autonomy and discretion.

ASSESSING PERFORMANCE

Defining performance indicators

If there is a unifying theme to performance measurement, then it lies in the genuflection to the objectives of economy, efficiency, and effectiveness, and to the production of measures of input, output, and outcome. These terms are common currency among practitioners and academics alike yet, as we saw in the previous chapter, there is considerable definitional and conceptual ambiguity regarding these two models. We cannot resolve all the confusions that pervade the literature but we will try to make them comprehensible. What we seek to do in the remainder of this chapter is to make our own models and assumptions explicit, to point out where we differ from other commentators, and to lay out the central problems that we will address in subsequent chapters.

We prefer to adopt a simple model which regards PIs in terms of inputs, processes, outputs, and outcomes. *Inputs* are the resources required to provide a service, including staff, buildings, equipment, and consumables. *Processes* are the way in which a service is delivered, and involves some measurement of quality, perhaps by inspectorates or via consumer complaints. *Outputs* are the activities of the organisation, or the service it provides, such as the number of benefit claims processed or patients treated (the terms 'throughput' and 'intermediate output' are frequently used instead of, or interchangeably with, 'output'). Finally, *outcome* is the impact of the service – healthier or more knowledgeable individuals, a safer society, and so on. This model and set of definitions is the one we shall work with but it is important to note that it is not universally accepted; some of the different versions used by recent contributors to the debate are illustrated in Table 2.2.

It is not always easy to determine whether these models reflect semantic or conceptual differences. To illustrate, Levitt and Joyce (1987) have constructed a hierarchy of outputs consisting of activities, intermediate outputs, and social consequences (or final outputs). Their conceptual distinctions mirror our own because 'consequences' are synonymous with our use of 'outcome' – 'poverty relieved, better health, improved knowledge, and less crime' (41) – i.e. it appears to be a simple

Table 2.2 A selection of alternative input–output models

INPUT	INPUT	INPUT	INPUT
PROCESS	OUTPUT	ACTIVITY	INTERMEDIATE OUTPUT
OUTPUT	IMPACT	THROUGHPUT CONSEQUENCE	THROUGHPUT OUTPUT OUTCOME
Butt and Palmer (1985) CIPFA (1984) HM Treasury (1986a, 1987)	Audit Commission (1986)	Levitt and Joyce (1987)	Flynn (1986)

semantic difference. But there may be a disguised conceptual difference because 'consequences' also appears to conflate outputs and outcomes: for example, exam results are regarded as proxy indicators of 'final output' (i.e. a consequence). But, using our schema, are exam results outputs or outcomes? Levitt and Joyce clearly use them as outcomes (and this is the way they are frequently used in practice), but we regard them as outputs; outcomes being a better educated, more skilled population (which may or may not be associated with exam results).

But there may be differences that reflect political perspectives; in the case of the Treasury model, the omission of any notion of outcome may indicate a reluctance to ask fundamental questions about the success of public policies, or an unwillingness or inability to define objectives against which performance can be assessed. On the other hand, as we saw in Chapter 1, it may be simply conceding that the technical problems of outcome measurement negate the utility of even making the attempt.

Although inputs and outputs used alone can provide some indication of performance, most organisations try to construct performance indicators that are based on ratios of inputs, outputs, and outcomes. In particular, the 'three Es' – economy, efficiency, and effectiveness – have gained wide currency at all levels of government during the 1980s because of the top-down pressure from the FMI and the Audit Commission to use this model. Yet some confusion also remains over the precise use of these technical terms.

In practice, public sector managers tend to assess *economy* exclusively in terms of costs. Reflecting this, some writers view economy in terms of 'how actual input costs compare with planned or expected costs' (Jackson and Palmer 1988: 32) or, simpler still, just 'minimising resource consumption' (Flynn *et al.* 1988: 38). Yet this approach, by focusing on inputs, completely ignores the quality of the output, i.e. whether it is of an acceptable standard. Consequently, we prefer to define economy as the purchase and provision of services at the lowest possible cost consistent with a specified quality; something which in principle should be an objective of any public sector service.

Efficiency is the ratio of inputs to outputs, or the rate at which inputs are converted into outputs. Used in this way, efficiency can rightly be regarded as 'intrinsically a politically neutral concept' (Levitt and Joyce 1987: 164). However, difficulties arise because, in practice, people are concerned with the objective of improving efficiency and this is when political judgements are made. Thus the Treasury and Civil Service

Committee (1982) defined an efficient programme as one where 'the actual output of a programme should be secured with the least use of resources' (xxvi), and the Audit Commission defined efficiency as a 'specified volume and quality of service with the lowest level of resources capable of meeting that requirement' (1986: 8). Yet, as Sir Peter Middleton, Permanent Secretary at the Treasury, has noted, efficiency is a two-sided coin; 'Do you get the maximum output from a given input, or do you get a given output from a minimum input?' (PAC 1987). Implicit in this statement is the admission that the official use of efficiency is rather one-sided; it is a distinction that may reflect contrasting approaches, i.e. an emphasis on cost-cutting as against service expansion.

Finally, *effectiveness* is a concept that is fraught with ambiguity and confusion. The Treasury and Civil Service Committee's less than succinct definition of effectiveness 'is one where the intention of the programme is being achieved', where 'the intention, the operational objectives and the targets have been defined; that the targets adequately represent the objectives and the objectives the intention and that the outputs of the programme are equal to the targets' (Treasury and Civil Service Committee 1982: xxvi). An obvious problem with this approach is that it makes the highly optimistic assumption that objectives are definable and non-conflicting; a view which was criticised earlier. Further, placing a priority on the achievement of any one goal in isolation may have a detrimental effect on the pursuit of other, conflicting goals. Even putting such objectives aside, there is some 'neat side-stepping' in this and in the similar Treasury definition of effectiveness as 'the ratio of output to planned output' (Pollitt 1986), or 'how far output achieves government objectives' (Jackson and Palmer 1988: 31). Indeed, in practice effectiveness may mean no more than the achievement of targets (Flynn *et al.* 1988). These definitions limit effectiveness to an evaluation of outputs of specific programmes; there is no attempt to link outputs and outcomes, and no assessment of the overall policy aims.

It may be useful therefore to distinguish between administrative and policy effectiveness. Administrative effectiveness is illustrated by Social Security clearance and error rates which, as we shall see in Chapter 4, assess whether that organisation is effective in providing beneficiaries with a payment that is correctly and speedily delivered. In contrast, policy effectiveness is the extent to which policy impacts meet policy aims, normally measured by the relationship between outputs and outcomes, and in this instance depends on the success of social security in attaining the final objective of relieving poverty in specific groups. To circumvent this distinction, Flynn *et al.* (1988) propose restricting effectiveness to measuring the achievement of targets or objectives, and introducing a fourth 'E' – efficacy – to measure the impact of programmes on the community. While this may be a valid intellectual distinction, its adoption might increase the focus on administrative effectiveness and reduce the incentive to pursue 'efficacy'. So, it may be better to retain the broader definition of effectiveness; making clear when organisations do employ narrower definitions that focus on the achievement of programme objectives, or weaker still, just on targets.

Several writers, notably Pollitt (1986), suggest that this subord-ination of outcomes to outputs (and the broader emphasis on economy and efficiency rather than effectiveness) may reflect the political interest of a government that is primarily concerned with cost-cutting rather than performance evaluation. Whatever the truth in this argument, it is important to recognise that, as we saw in the previous chapter, the under-emphasis on effectiveness may also indicate the enormous technical problem of establishing the causal relationship between outputs and outcome. On this point, it is worth noting the Audit Commission's barbed criticism of 'academic critics' who berate the Commission for ignoring effectiveness 'without being particularly clear about what this might mean in practice or how it could be reconciled with the Commission's lack of standing on policy issues' (1986: para. 7b).

The 'three Es' model has further limitations, one of which is its narrow focus. Several observers have proposed additional 'Es': efficacy, electability (Flynn *et al.* 1988), and equity (ibid.; Pollitt 1986); or extensions to the alphabet of performance such as acceptability and availability (Clarke 1984). This list could undoubtedly keep growing but as it is not our intention at this stage to debate all the possible dimensions of performance measurement, we will discuss here only what is probably the most important, and most discussed, alternative: equity.

An important (perhaps defining) characteristic of the public sector is the expectation that due process will be exercised in the delivery of services. Equity, or administrative justice, implies that in all similar cases individuals will be dealt with alike, within the terms set by the law. This suggests that equity should be a bottom-line PI for any public service. The recent emphasis upon the 'three Es' and, in particular, the pressure to improve efficiency may have implications for equity: put simply, will the achievement of greater efficiency be at the cost of equity? For example, it may be possible to shuffle money through the social security system more quickly and hence more efficiently, but this may be achieved at the cost of providing a poorer service to claimants who may have to wait longer in the office or have less time with officials because staff have been relocated to other activities. Clearly it is important to monitor and maintain equity in the delivery of public sector services.

But equity is a difficult word to define. We have used it in its narrowest form – due process or administrative justice – but it can have wider applications. There can be equity in policy-making in the sense of neutrality and fairness as between different groups, or equity defined as positive discrimination in favour of disadvantaged groups such as women and ethnic minorities; this broader political definition has found greatest favour in the USA (Rivlin 1971). This conceptual ambiguity makes it difficult to incorporate equity into the 'three Es' model.

A more serious objection arises from an odd omission from the discussion of performance assessment. Quite simply, the literature on performance indicators ignores the machinery that is specifically designed to protect equity. This 'forgotten' constitutional machinery consists of a range of instruments that includes the parliamentary question, the various species of local and national ombudsmen and administrative tribunals. To take but one example, as we shall see in Chapter 4 in the Department of Social Security there is a Social Security Commissioner, appeals tribunals, and a Chief Adjudication Officer (Sainsbury 1989) which, in different ways, all exist for the redress of individual grievances. Other departments have similar institutional arrangements. We do not suggest that these formal instruments are necessarily sufficient for ensuring equity – Social Security, say, might benefit from monitoring claimant complaints more carefully. But it does suggest that PIs are only one part of the process for ensuring equity. We need to ask what relationship exists between the instruments for the redress of individual grievances and the mechanisms for performance assessment. Indeed, is there any relationship? If not, ought there to be? It is because of this overlap with other constitutional arrangements that we choose not to incorporate equity into the 'three Es' model. This is not to deny the importance of equity; rather it is to argue that equity should play a supplementary as opposed to a central role in any model of PIs.

A further criticism of the PIs generated by the 'three Es' model is that they tend to ignore the quality aspect of service delivery (North East Thames RHA 1984; Pollitt 1986, 1987a). Yet concepts like efficiency are predicated on the maintenance of constant quality: any improvement in efficiency should not be at the expense of quality of service. Also, any evaluation of process is heavily dependent on an assessment of quality. Thus it is clearly important to monitor quality. However, there are methodological problems in measuring quality because, unlike technical concepts such as efficiency, it is often difficult to quantify what constitutes good quality in terms of, say, policing or health provision. But where there is a definable product such as money or water then it is less difficult to construct quality measures. As we saw in Chapter 1, caseload departments like Inland Revenue and Social Security simply find it both conceptually and technically easier to construct PIs that measure the speed and accuracy of service, i.e. quality. Yet as we shall see in Chapter 4, even in caseload departments like Social Security, there is great uncertainty about what quality actually is and how it can be measured. This suggests that the organisational dimension is significant in the production of quality PIs, and it is a theme to which we shall return in the final chapter.

The issue of quality raises a linked question about the role of consumers in performance evaluation. It has been argued that the perceptions of the consumer are an essential part of measuring both quality and effectiveness (National Consumer Council 1986; Pollitt 1988). After all, it is consumers or clients who are on the receiving end of service delivery and, so the argument goes, surely only they can decide whether the service is providing them with the quality of processes and volume of outputs that they want? This is particularly pertinent for many public sector services which are monopoly providers and therefore offer consumers no exit opportunities; in this context, consumers should be given every opportunity for voice. However, amongst the coalition of interests that make up public sector organisations there are various groups that may be opposed to listening to the consumer: for example, politicians may dislike any challenge to their particular view of the service, and managers may be keen to defend their managerial prerogative to make decisions. Most important, the agenda-setting professional service providers have every incentive to resist any incursion by the consumer on their autonomy. Moreover, consumers may be fearful of victimisation if they do exercise voice, particularly if they make a complaint about police behaviour or ask for a second medical opinion. Thus, whether public sector monopolies do listen to consumers may depend on the influence of external political pressures persuading them to do so. In other words, will the political market – in the form of pressure from parliamentary institutions such as the National Audit Office, Select Committees, etc. – substitute for the competitive market which brings its own pressures to provide what the consumers want? This brief discussion of the consumer dimension has raised questions rather than provided answers, and will be explored further in subsequent chapters.

PUTTING PERFORMANCE INDICATORS TO USE

Underlying much discussion about PIs is a degree of confusion about the precise role that they are performing in organisations, for PIs have a variety of uses depending on their purpose and location in each organisation. They can be used to monitor the overall strategic or operational performance of the organisation, as an instrument of hands-off control over the lower levels of the organisation, as a tool for day-to-day management by the street-level bureaucrat, or they can form part of the process of individual appraisal and in allocating performance related pay. And they can be used by many different actors: obviously managers (at several different levels), but also by national and local politicians, professionals, consumers, and even the workforce; clearly, there is a wealth of interest in PIs (Pollitt 1986).

This eclecticism may have an impact on the design of PI systems. The existence of multiple constituencies *within* organisations (quite apart from *external* stakeholders) means that different constituencies will actively prefer different definitions of performance, and hence advocate different measures. Kanter and Summers (1987) drew the following conclusion from their study of non-profit organisations:

> Managers might prefer structural measures of organisational characteristics because they have control over such factors; the rank and file might prefer process measures of activities because they control their own performance; and clients and customers prefer outcome measures because they want results, not promises or mere effort.
>
> (158)

This suggests the importance of asking the following questions of any organisation: who wants PIs, who uses them, and why?

However, there have been very few attempts comprehensively to classify PIs according to the roles they perform. One example is Pollitt's (1987b) typology based on three organisational mechanisms: whether the scheme is compulsory or voluntary, whether it is linked to a formal incentive scheme, and whether it evaluates individual or organisational performance. In particular, Pollitt distinguishes management-driven 'efficiency from above' schemes which are characterised by hierarchy, competitiveness, and the 'right to manage', from self-driven professional models. Clearly, these two ideal types will profoundly differ in their objectives, their application, and the form they take. However, although it isolates important themes, this taxonomy is limited as an explanatory tool because most public sector PI packages fit the same category; being compulsory, measuring organisational performance, and having no links with formal incentive schemes (though this may change with the influx of performance related pay schemes).

In contrast to this all-embracing approach, other studies have concentrated on specific uses of PIs. For example, Carter (1989) argues that the FMI has encouraged senior managers to use PIs as an instrument of 'hands-off' control but that this objective encounters a series of obstacles that have frequently resulted in PIs being regarded as an unwanted form of 'backseat driving'. Alternatively, as we have already seen, others have focused on the consumer as the forgotten dimension of performance evaluation (Pollitt 1988; National Consumer Council 1986).

Further clues may be found in the way that PIs are used differently according to the level at which they operate within an organisation. An area or regional manager may possess and use detailed information about individual branch performance, but the figures that reach national level management may not be open to disaggregation: for example, until recent changes in the law, local education authority PIs were not disaggregated to the level of individual schools, and were not generally available to the Department of Education and Science. If the technology and information is available – which is not always the case – why is a more detailed picture not required? In the case of education, the autonomy enjoyed by local education authorities (LEAs) and their arm's-length relationship with the DES provided the organisational explanation; the fear of publicising the performance of individual schools (due to parental reaction) a further political reason. But it could be that senior management will often not need (or want) greater detail because it is only concerned with monitoring performance at a strategic level; it is up to area or regional managers to monitor the performance of sub-units or of individuals.

In practice it may not be at all clear what purpose PIs are serving; indeed, they are likely to be filling more than one role. Consequently, it may be useful to shift our focus slightly in order to ask what factors influence the effectiveness of PIs – whatever their purpose might be. But what makes a good PI? There is no definitive answer to this question, although various commentators have suggested the basic criteria that a PI system should satisfy (see Cave *et al.* 1988; Jackson 1988). We have already touched on a number of factors. Definitions must be clear and consistent. A PI should measure performance that is 'owned' by the organisation and not dependent on external actors or environmental factors. Others are common sense. PIs should be relevant to the needs and objectives of the organisation. They should not be susceptible to manipulation by the person or unit to be assessed, such as the infamous 'citation circles' formed by academics to boost one another's citation level when this PI is used as an indicator of the standard of research (Cave *et al.* 1988).

Not every characteristic is uncontroversial. Thus Jackson suggests that PI schemes should be both 'comprehensive' (reflecting all those aspects of behaviour that are critical to managerial decision-making) and 'bounded' (concentrating on a limited number of PIs). The preference for 'boundedness' stems from the widespread concern in many public sector organisations about the sheer volume of PIs. A system with a large number of PIs may be unwieldy; practitioners often bemoan the cost of collecting and monitoring PIs which arguably negates any savings arising from their use. But is parsimony compatible with an evaluation system that embraces all aspects of performance? Boundedness may provide only a partial picture of overall performance, focusing on certain aspects and ignoring others. Can these contradictions be reconciled? Here we might speculate that the more heterogeneous an organisation, the greater the number of PIs. Complexity might also point in this direction, particularly if different professions or occupational groups in an organisation insist on their own, autonomous definition of performance.

One of the most important attributes of any PI is the credibility of the information upon which it is built, i.e. how accurate and comprehensive is the database? If the information is unreliable then many of the criteria of PIs will be impossible to achieve. Significantly, many public sector organisations have been forced by a combination of political pressures (notably MINIS and the FMI) and operating circumstances to make major investments in information technology (Beard 1988). This is crucial because information technology is a critical enabling factor in the emergence of a sophisticated PI system. For the quality of information has conceptual implications for the design and use of PIs; put simply, the data dictate what can be measured. This point is well illustrated by the question of timeliness: how often are PIs produced? In practice, PIs are often generated slowly and infrequently, perhaps some months after the event. As a result the figures may be 'history' by the time they are produced, bearing little relevance to contemporary problems. This affects the use to which PIs can be put; without up-to-date accurate data the potential for immediate trouble-shooting or redeployment of resources by management is limited. Speculating again, we might expect the speed of production to depend on the sensitivity of the organisation to external pressures (e.g. market competition) and its steerability (whether or not it responds quickly to touches on the wheel). Last, a critical factor is the extent to which the flow and accessibility of information throughout an organisation is enhanced by the use of modern information technology: in the 1960s, there was one large computer generating information at headquarters; today, in most organisations, every manager has access to their own terminal. This not only helps to improve the two-way vertical flow of information, it also enhances and encourages the use of PIs at all levels of the organisation.

All the above characteristics of the PI contribute to a more subjective dimension; namely the acceptability of PIs by the members of the organisation. We can illustrate this point by recalling Pollitt's (1987b) taxonomy: a bottom-up, peer review scheme might be attractive to employees, but a scheme imposed on the workforce may be treated with great suspicion, provoking a response similar to the dreaded factory time-and-motion study, i.e. PIs will be seen as an instrument of management control that may lead to wage cuts, an increased workload, or even redundancies. It is worth recalling that the resistance of trade unions during the early 1970s contributed to the early termination of a number of Management By Objectives and performance measurement schemes in the DHSS (Garrett 1980). Consequently, returning to the issue of information, it seems reasonable to suggest that no amount of advanced technology will ever produce a uniformly acceptable PI system because acceptability is as much a political as a technical concept. If organisations consist of multiple constituencies there will probably always be at least one group willing to pick holes in a data set; ultimately the credibility of information may reside in the eye of the beholder.

Thus acceptability is a complex notion. The acceptance of PIs (in the sense of acquiescence) is at best only a first step towards incorporating PIs in the culture and life of the organisation whereby individuals internalise a different way of thinking. Many managers talk about the 'psychology' involved in introducing this kind of organisational change; certainly the culture of the organisation may alter substantially. In short, the successful introduction of PIs is contingent on the availability of appropriate managerial skills, a very considerable investment of effort at all levels of management, and the development of PIs that are meaningful to staff. If PIs are not grounded in the everyday work of the individual members of staff, they will be dismissed as irrelevant and may prove an unwieldy, arbitrary, and divisive organisational tool with the costs outweighing the benefits. Acceptability may also depend on the existence of the necessary incentives to use PIs. Incentives may vary from being directly instrumental such as when PIs are built into a system of individual appraisal or performance related pay, to having an indirect organisational pay-off where PIs are regarded by certain constituencies as a means of exercising greater power or, more generally, as a tool for obtaining increased external funding for the service.

One vital question remains: what gives 'meaning' to PIs? How can PIs be used to evaluate 'good' and 'bad' performance when there are no explicit standards? Relativity plagues most of the service organisations studied in this book: for example, if crime levels are indicators of performance then what is an acceptable level of crime? What is a 'reasonable' waiting period for an operation to remove varicose veins, for a Crown Court case to be heard, or for claimants to receive benefits? Relativity particularly besets organisations that pursue multiple and contradictory objectives or where the ownership of performance lies beyond the boundaries of the organisation. However, what we fall back on is an acceptance that standard-setting is a political process involving a complex mix of financial, social, technical, and historical criteria for assessing performance.

In practice, managers try to overcome these problems by starting from the assumption that the performance of an organisational unit must be compared on a like-with-like basis, i.e. between units that carry out similar functions with a broadly similar population. But this is not always easy: if the currency of assessment is comparison with other units, how do we know that like is being compared with like? Is it fair or useful to compare the performance of a large inner city Social Security office with that of a small rural office? Or a London hospital with a cottage hospital? A high security prison with a remand centre? Consequently, several types of comparison are employed in an attempt to circumvent or reduce the problems of like-with-like and variable case-mix:

1 *Targets*: the analysis of performance against the achievement of policy or budgeting targets is widespread; Bexley Council (1985) boasts a particularly large set of targets across a wide range of services. Target-setting avoids the problem of like-for-like, but raises questions about the process of selecting targets. Who decides the targets: are they imposed from above, do they emerge from below, or are they negotiated between levels? Are the targets realistic? Are they linked to incentive schemes?

2 *Time-series*: comparison with the historical record of the same organisation. In theory the time-series overcomes the problem of like-for-like comparison but in practice many variables are liable to change. The introduction of new technology can transform the operation of a service, particularly those involving the dissemination of information or the provision of benefits. Changes to the quality of information due to new technology will make the time-series

redundant (or else the time-series will not be updated and hence become unreliable). Demographic or social changes may alter the demand for a service: falling school rolls may force the closure of schools; an ageing population will require more residential homes. Exceptional circumstances influence the performance of a service in a particular year; a strike by teachers or a year of drought may create a 'blip' in the performance figures for education and water supply. There are also problems about the 'validity' of the benchmark. If performance was previously inefficient then the introduction of PIs may produce a remarkable improvement, whereas an already excellent record may present little scope for improvement. Moreover, when PIs are first designed the actual data may be unreliable or even non-existent.

3 *Comparable Organisational Units*: a cross-sectional comparison with other units of the same service, often leading to 'league tables'. This may occur at a variety of levels: the recent exercise carried out by the Universities Funding Council (1989) permitted the ranking of academic departments according to discipline, of small groupings of departments based on 'cost centres', and even of an overall average for each university. Clearly, many of the organisational dimensions discussed above come into play here. How can a variable case-mix be accommodated when comparing apparently similar units? Comparing university departments in terms of research and publications may ignore significant differences in teaching and administrative loads which will influence the amount of time free for staff to undertake research. If sub-units and universities are compared in terms of research income generated, then some disciplines will benefit over others because they are in a position to attract more funds than others: medical research receives more money than philosophy. Consequently, the mix of disciplines will influence the performance of the larger unit. More generally, should different socio-economic features be taken into account? Returning to an earlier example, should exam performance be analysed on a simple results basis as the government has done (*Hansard* 12/2/85) or should an adjustment be made for variables like class background and ethnic origins? One solution to this is some form of cluster analysis: the Audit Commission and CIPFA have both constructed lists of 'nearest neighbour' or 'family' local authorities with a similar socio-economic profile (see also Webber and Craig 1976). This can be used as a precise statistical model or as a 'rough and ready' (CIPFA 1984) comparison with the option of pursuing a case study approach in different units (Hill and Bramley 1986).

4 *External Comparison*: it is possible to look at the performance of
   other organisations, both public and private, although this option is
   not yet used widely. The key question here again is like-for-like: how
   far can a comparison of banks and social security offices be taken?
   Flynn (1986) argues that the only readily transferable measures are
   those referring to unit cost of inputs (gross hourly rates) or from
   within the production function (percentage of administrative,
   professional, technical staff), but this seems unduly restrictive.
   Indeed, Levitt and Joyce (1987) make some interesting productivity
   comparisons between the staff–client ratios of clearing banks,
   building societies, Customs and Excise, and the Inland Revenue, and
   the cost ratios of life insurance companies, Customs and Excise, the
   Inland Revenue, and Social Security. Their (fascinating) conclusion,
   subject to a number of caveats, concerns 'the degree of similarity
   between the government departments and private financial
   institutions ... despite significant differences in the financial
   incentives to the staff concerned. This is not to say that either or both
   are maximising their potential' (66).

There is also a danger that average performance will be equated with
good performance. It might be that, in practice, PIs direct attention to
statistical outliers, i.e. those units or branches that appear to be
performing extraordinarily badly. But it is one thing to say that this is a
valid 'signal for inquiry', and quite another thing to presume that it is
necessarily the worst performer. How can it be assumed that those
'hiding in the pack' are, by definition, performing well and that no
questions need to be asked about them? And what happens after a
period of time when PIs have been used to 'bring in' the outliers thereby
compressing performance? How are PIs to be used then? These
questions are all the more critical because of the problem of
heterogeneity. If the product itself is heterogeneous (as in the case of the
NHS) then which dimensions of performance count for how much?
What is the rate of exchange for the different PI currencies? Moreover,
what if there is geographical heterogeneity? If PIs are being used to
assess an agency delivering services through a variety of outlets – be it a
district health authority or a local education authority – then is the sum
of its performance the only relevant factor, or should this be broken
down into its components parts? For example, there are many schools
in an LEA and an average figure giving exam performance or average
cost per pupil may conceal a wide disparity of performances: there could
be one or two centres of excellence carrying the rest, or there could be a
consistent average across all the schools.

Thus there are a number of techniques that are employed to circumvent or lessen the problem of relativity. But they do not avoid the underlying dilemma that without normative standards PIs will constantly come up against the issue of what makes 'good' and 'bad' performance; in many organisations this will remain an unresolvable problem. However, to help distinguish the main uses of PIs in a way that directly addresses the question of standards, we have adopted a simple conceptual scheme that classifies the use of PIs as either prescriptive, descriptive, or proscriptive.

Prescriptive PIs are those which, in the classic style of proposed reforms of management in government from Fulton to FMI, are linked to objectives or targets. Ministers or managers set the objectives and the PIs are subsequently used to monitor progress towards their achievement. In contrast, *descriptive* PIs simply record change: they provide a map rather than a prescribed route through the terrain. Lastly, *proscriptive* or negative PIs specify not targets or ends but things which simply should not happen in a well-run organisation.

To clarify these three categories of PI it may be helpful to think of PIs as being used either as dials, tin-openers, or alarm-bells. Obviously, from the point of view of controlling service delivery and ease of use, the ideal prescriptive PI operates like a dial, providing a precise measure of inputs, outputs, and outcomes based on a clear understanding of what good and bad performance entails. But public sector organisations have very few precise measures; one example would be the water authorities where they can measure the number of overflowing sewers against an explicit normative standard. Similarly, the electricity industry's measures of the number of minutes of electricity supply lost per customer per year or the percentage of repairs successfully completed on the first visit are PIs that can be read off like a dial and judged against normative standards (Electricity Council 1988). However, PIs are frequently used prescriptively without having clear standards for assessing performance. For example, departments are increasingly adopting a target-setting approach: as Lord Young has observed, the advantage of target PIs like 'ten per cent of teachers by 1990 to spend some time in industry each year' (*The Independent* 7/3/88) is that they are at least measurable, if less precise than a normative measure of water quality.

In practice, PIs tend to be used descriptively. Most PIs are tin-openers rather than dials: by opening up a 'can of worms' they do not give answers but prompt interrogation and inquiry, and by themselves provide an incomplete and inaccurate picture. For example, if an academic researcher receives a high number of citations this may be a mark of respected scholarship, or it may be that the academic has published one or two poor and controversial articles in a widely researched field which every other researcher is simply obliged to refer to . . . if only to condemn and dismiss! Clearly, citation indexes do not provide answers, the figures can only start an argument. Implicit in the use of PIs as dials is the assumption that standards of performance are unambiguous; implicit in the use of PIs as tin-openers is the assumption that performance is a contestable notion.

A PI may be value-laden but not directly prescriptive; that is, it may include a presumption that a movement in a particular direction – such as towards lower unit costs or lower error rates – is desirable, without setting a specific target. Here the emphasis is on travelling along a particular route rather than arriving at a specified destination; it is about comparing relative performance over time, rather than performance against normative standards or precise targets.

The third category, the proscriptive PI, operates like an alarm-bell, by giving warning that things are happening which should not be tolerated in a well-run organisation. Of course, there may be an overlap here. The negative PI can also be used both prescriptively, setting a target for flooding sewers, and descriptively, monitoring and analysing consumer complaints. Although there are many negative PIs in the public sector the idea is rarely given explicit recognition, despite the conceptual precedents contained in the maternal deaths inquiry in the NHS as long ago as 1967 (DHSS 1972).

The different uses given to PIs have implications for management styles, even though many services may use a mix of dials and tin-openers. The prescriptive PI will generally be a top-down management tool that lends itself to a command style of management. But if performance cannot be read off a dial, if comparisons are problematic, how do different organisations handle the negotiations and bargaining involved in determining what excuses are acceptable? Thus the descriptive PI, which can be produced at any level of the organisation, suggests the need for a more persuasive style of management; far from being a simple top-down exercise, performance assessment instead necessarily involves a complicated and often highly political process of negotiation at and between different levels of management and activity.

One conclusion, above all, stands out from both the history of managerial reforms discussed in Chapter 1 and the review of the main concepts and issues in the performance literature. This is that the notion of performance – often bereft of normative standards, invariably full of ambiguity – is, in theory and practice, both contestable and complex. It seems apparent that differences between organisations and the nature of service delivery will profoundly influence the design and use of PIs; in other words, the problems of performance assessment transcend the public/private dichotomy. The commonly held belief that performance assessment differs between public and private organisations because the latter possess the bottom line, profit, does not stand up to examination.

In our case studies we explore our hunch that it is a set of organisational characteristics as much as the conventional public/private divide which may best explain how performance is assessed in practice. In so doing, we draw on the experience of a number of private sector service organisations. A plethora of questions come to mind. Where does the searchlight of assessment fall? Does it fall on inputs, processes, outputs, or outcomes? Will we find significant differences between public and private sector organisations? Given the absence of a bottom line which makes the measurement of effectiveness so difficult, will we find public sector organisations concentrating more on process than private sector organisations? How do private organisations overcome the problems of relative standards? Of comparing like with like? Of measuring quality of service delivery? The following chapters provide some of the answers to these and other questions.

3 The criminal justice system
Police, courts, and prisons

This chapter examines three organisations that make up the core elements of the criminal justice system in England and Wales but which, in practice, face very different problems in assessing organisational performance: they are the Police, the Lord Chancellor's Department, and the Prison Service.

THE POLICE

The performance of the police, of all the organisations examined in this book, has probably been the subject of most public criticism and political controversy in recent years. Whether this is due to the apparently inexorable increase in crime levels, the policing of Poll Tax demonstrations or strikes at Wapping, the acquittal of the Guildford Four, the allegations concerning the West Midlands Crime Squad or the Stalker affair *inter alia*, the competence and integrity of the service has been widely questioned. This often hostile criticism has prompted a wide-ranging political debate about ways of increasing police accountability. Yet, despite this pressure to account for police performance, progress in developing PIs or any other means of scrutinising its performance has been amongst the slowest of the organisations covered in this study.

Policing in England and Wales is carried out predominantly within the public sector. The combined total of all police forces and units represents a large organisation consisting of 124,856 officers and 47,234 civilians in 1989 (HM Treasury 1990: Cmnd. 1009). It is in a monopoly position with the exception of private detective agencies and a private security police industry concerned with the protection of property (the mushrooming of the latter may represent an interesting PI of police performance). The police is also primarily a non-trading organisation – although it does charge for certain services, such as the policing of football stadiums – the police budget being shared almost equally between central and local government.

In theory, there is no single body that can be called 'the police': the forty-three police forces in England and Wales are all separate organisations tied to local government. Each force is governed by a tripartite arrangement. Briefly: the chief constable directs and controls the individual force; the police authority, consisting of county councillors and magistrates, is responsible for the 'adequacy and efficiency' of the force and it has amongst its powers the right to appoint the chief constable; finally, the Home Secretary is charged with promoting the efficiency of the police and possesses significant powers, including control over 51 per cent of the budget of each force (ibid.), the use of the Inspectorate of Constabulary, the right to veto the choice of a chief constable, and direct control over the Metropolitan police – the largest single force in England and Wales. This complex structure is at odds with clear lines of political accountability and enables the chief constable to exercise considerable *de facto* autonomy. However, it is widely accepted that in recent years the Home Office has increased its control over the police so that police policy is largely determined by the centre: no more is it a politically controlled local service, instead 'policing has become more a national service which is administered locally' (Morgan 1987: 75). Despite this, although policing is no more than a 'self-defined' profession, as a group the police reserves the right to have its performance judged only by its peers; a level of autonomy also enjoyed by judges and doctors, as we describe later in the book.

The police ranks in the middle category for heterogeneity because, although it serves a wide variety of client groups it does not have an enormous range of discrete products in terms of the variety of activities pursued by its officers. Hence the police can be categorised as low on organisational complexity because, as the figures above indicate, the vast majority of its establishment consists of a single-skill labour force.

In contrast, the police is very high on uncertainty because of its multiple objectives and because of the very tenuous relationship between outputs and outcomes. The police service has to pursue a myriad of objectives which include traffic control, the maintenance of law and order, community relations, crime prevention, and the control of drug trafficking. These objectives frequently conflict: for example, a heavy police presence at a football match or at a music festival may deter fighting on the streets or catch a few drug dealers but possibly at the cost of good community relations. Individual functions also have multiple objectives: Sinclair and Miller (1984) have pointed to 'the difficulty of defining what the police and patrolling police officers are trying to do and of determining how much of their time they devote to one purpose rather than another' (14). Is the purpose of patrol to prevent crime, maintain public order, improve community relations, or what? It is also very difficult to isolate cause and effect between police activity and outcome. For example, crime levels are clearly influenced by a number of environmental factors over which the police has no control: economic factors such as unemployment or social factors such as drinking or drug taking may all have an impact on crime levels. The police therefore faces a particularly perplexing problem of performance ownership that, amongst all our organisations, is matched only by the uncertainty characterising the delivery of health care.

The design and use of performance indicators in the police

The police is a public service steeped in the tradition that good performance depends primarily on inputs and processes illustrated by, for example, the still widely held belief that there is a direct relationship between the number of officers and the impact on crime, and the notion of the kindly, observable, 'bobby on the beat'. There has always been an interest in improving operational efficiency: the move from foot patrols to the vehicle-based Unit Beat Policing in the late-1960s was based on the assumption that this would cut down response times and hence improve good relations with the public (it was the perceived failure to achieve this objective that led to a limited return to foot patrol during the 1980s) (Weatheritt 1986). There was also a short-lived attempt to improve financial efficiency when, between 1969 and 1974, the Home Office introduced Planning, Programming, Budgeting (PPBS) into twelve forces. PPBS involved organising police expenditure into a series of functional categories with the ultimate aim of developing output measures based on these functions so that a relationship between cost and performance could be established (see Christian 1982). When the Home Office withdrew support in 1974, individual forces abandoned PPBS because they perceived few benefits from the new costing system. In particular, there was dissatisfaction that central government was able neither to specify precise policing objectives nor to construct useful measures of police performance (Weatheritt 1986).

Before the 1980s the police had never come under political pressure from central government to construct 'objective' measures of performance. There was a cross-party consensus supporting the police that avoided any involvement in internal police matters: indeed, rising crime levels in the 1970s persuaded the Callaghan Administration to divert more resources to the police and the election of the Thatcher

Administration, committed to law and order, heralded a period of unprecedented growth in expenditure on the police. As a result, staffing levels rose 11 per cent between 1978 and 1982, and pay was increased by 16 per cent in real terms in the four years to 1984. Thus the police consistently obtained extra resources to 'put more bobbies on the beat', without providing any evidence about the effectiveness of the extra officers.

Slowly, however, the profligacy of police spending began to meet the disapproving eye of a government that was also anxious to contain public expenditure and increasingly concerned about the lack of observable improvement in police performance. There was a growing recognition in government that 'the traditional "holy trinity" response of more powers, more equipment, and more manpower has not substantially impacted on the problem' (Jones and Silverman 1984: 34). It was not simply a matter of cost-cutting; the Government was increasingly sceptical about the effectiveness of policing methods. As Sir Brian Cubbon, Under-Secretary of State at the Home Office, said in evidence to the Public Accounts Committee, '. . .you are getting more bobbies on the beat. But there is a further question(s) which lies behind that which is: what are they doing? . . . what are we getting for the money?' (1987: 30). One manifestation of the changing approach was the decision to hold police numbers level during the period 1982–6; another was the publication of Home Office Circular 114/1983 *Manpower, Effectiveness and Efficiency in the Police Service.*

Circular 114/83 represented the official response to the FMI. The message was clear: this was a statement of the Home Office's intention to improve efficiency and effectiveness allied to constraints on police expenditure. It provided a new framework for all forces to follow when seeking an increase in their establishment: in contrast to the years of almost unrestrained expansion, a chief constable now had to make a specific case for extra staff.

Chief constables were expected to establish precise objectives and priorities which had to be communicated to all levels of the force; subsequently, a list of objectives and priorities was included in the annual report of each chief constable. The emphasis on objective-setting was more than a knee-jerk response to the FMI; there was also a widespread concern within the service about the lack of objectives. This was but one strand of a broader internal debate about police management in which many commentators were advocating the introduction of more rational managerial techniques involving improved management information and the use of performance measures (Collins 1985). In particular, there was great interest in the strategy of 'Policing by Objectives' (PBO) which has been enthusiastically endorsed by

Butler (1985), implicitly recommended in Circular 114/1983, and since implemented by some forty forces (Joint Consultative Committee 1990).

The circular was more reticent about fulfilling the second part of the FMI policy requiring 'the means to assess, and wherever possible measure, outputs or performance in relation to those objectives'. Although it employed the language of rational management – 'objectives', 'priorities', 'efficiency' were all prominent – and stressed the need for forces to review police policies and performance regularly, the circular contained no detailed plans to develop a system of performance indicators.

There were of course various existing indicators that could be used to assess police performance: a wide number of statistics about police and criminal activity were and are available in two annual Home Office publications: the *Report of HM Inspector of Constabulary* and **Criminal Statistics**. The only PIs listed in the Public Expenditure White Paper are the crime rate (the number of recorded notifiable offences) and the clear-up rate (the number of notifiable offences cleared up). These figures are disaggregated for specific offences – crimes of violence notified and cleared up are monitored with particular concern – and into an overall 'productivity' indicator – the number of offences cleared up per officer (see Table 3.1). Although these statistics receive widespread media coverage, crime levels and clear-up rates have been widely

Table 3.1 Notifiable offences recorded and cleared up

	1984	1985	1986	1987	1988
Notifiable offences:					
recorded (000s)	3,314	3,426	3,660	3,716	3,550
cleared up (000s)	1,150	1,212	1,157	1,229	1,249
Clear-up rate (all notifiable offences) (per cent)	35	35	32	33	35
Notifiable offences per officer:					
recorded	27.4	28.4	30.2	30.2	28.5
cleared up	9.5	10.1	9.5	9.9	10.0
Offences of violence against the person:					
recorded (000s)	114.2	121.7	125.5	141.0	158.2
cleared up (000s)	84.0	88.5	89.5	105.1	119.4
Clear-up rate (offences of violence against the person) (per cent)	74	73	71	75	75

Source: HM Treasury (1990), Cmnd. 1009

criticised by practitioners and academics alike as representing very poor indicators of police effectiveness.

There are problems with the quality of the figures and with what they represent in terms of police performance. First, what do crime levels tell us about the pervasiveness of crime? Home Office surveys reveal that the official crime rate seriously underestimates the true level of crime. Many crimes are never reported: perhaps because an effective response is presumed unlikely, or because victims take alternative means of resolving a problem, perhaps taking the law into their own hands. On the other hand, in *Criminal Statistics*, the Home Office suggests that a large part of the increase in the official crime rate is due to the greater propensity of victims to report crime, rather than reflecting a rise in the actual level of crime. Explanations of this include greater telephone ownership, wider insurance cover, better recording practices, and changing public attitudes, although the last two lack empirical support (Harrison and Gretton 1986). There is also evidence suggesting that recorded crime rises with an increase in the number of police officers.

Second, chief constables frequently disown responsibility for crime figures that apparently reflect poor police performance: Sir Kenneth Newman, then Chief Constable of the Metropolitan Police, deflected criticism about large increases in London crime figures during 1986 by pointing to the impact of environmental factors on crime levels: 'Figures that are supposed to be performance measures of the police are in fact a performance measure of society as a whole'. Similarly, detection rates may not reflect efficient investigative effort on the part of the police but simply 'chance' factors such as 'immediate identification by victims or witnesses, offences admitted to be "taken into consideration" or admitted during follow-up visits to offenders in prison' (Reiner 1988: 33). Of these figures the most useful is the clear-up rate per officer which at least raises questions such as why the clear-up rate has remained constant at about 9.5 per cent per officer over a period in which the police benefited from extra staff, new technology, and improved training. Significantly the White Paper warns that the figures 'must be interpreted with caution' (HM Treasury 1990: Cmnd. 1009).

In the face of the problems associated with using crime figures as an overall indicator of police effectiveness and the lack of less ambitious PIs that could be used to assess operational efficiency and effectiveness, it is perhaps surprising that circular 114/1983 did not impose any central direction on the development of PIs, leaving it instead to the initiative of individual forces to construct their own. This reluctance to assume responsibility probably reflected the need to pacify chief constables worried about further encroachment on their autonomy. This policy of encouraging a bottom-up approach clearly failed: a recent review carried out by the Joint Consultative Committee (1990) of the three Police Staff Associations in England and Wales admitted that: 'in retrospect, the police service failed to grasp this opportunity of fully developing its own rigorous measures of performance'. More specifically, this report discovered that even as late as 1989 twenty-seven forces (almost two-thirds) were unable to supply basic quantitative performance measures, observing wryly that 'this might be thought surprising given the requirements of the earlier circular 114'. Of those forces that had made some effort to respond to circular 114, there were a wide variety of initiatives including activity analysis, workload analysis, public opinion surveys, professional judgement, and the construction of matrices of statistics. Clearly, without guidance and direction there has been duplication of effort, confusion, and a lack of the uniformity needed to allow comparison between forces. In short, it was an excellent example of the centre/periphery tension that characterises the police as an organisation.

However, although the Home Office did not use circular 114 to impose any central system on individual forces, it did take a lead in improving police management systems. Clearly, the FMI provided an opportunity to develop systems that would allow the centre to exercise greater control over individual police forces. Initially, progress was slow and hindered by various technical and organisational problems. For example, an early Home Office-sponsored research study was unable to isolate many credible or useful performance measures (Sinclair and Miller 1984) but eventually it was decided to give the Inspectorate of Constabulary the primary responsibility for developing PIs. Two major initiatives were launched: first, the construction of a 'financial information system' based on a system of functional costing; second, the development of a set of functional statistics recording police activity called the 'matrix of indicators'.

The aim of the financial information system was to enable costings to be matched with activities and outputs. The system allocated costs to eight functional categories of activities: the operational activities were patrol, crime, traffic, public order, community relations, and others; the non-operational activities were training and management. This generated data over time which were an improvement on annual establishment returns that provided a mere snapshot of a particular moment.

The system was piloted in several forces during 1983 and 1984, but several problems were uncovered; notably as over half of police activity was taken up by the one functional category of 'patrol' it was necessary to disaggregate this function. But the construction of efficiency measures proved a problem. For example, the efficiency indicator for patrol was 'cost per incident response' yet responding to incidents is not the sole purpose of patrol; for example, there is also the preventive element. Moreover, a force could double its so-called efficiency at a stroke, simply by halving the numbers on patrol; but is this efficient? Similarly, the efficiency indicator for complaints was 'cost per complaint received', but this took no account of how complaints were resolved. The most 'efficient' force would not investigate complaints! The designers also faced difficulties in standardising recording practices between forces. There were many similar problems that contributed to the financial information system failing to win favour in Home Office circles. The system clearly received low priority; officials complained about the absence of qualified staff allocated to police costings, 'I am astounded by the lack of administrative staff on the budgeting side of affairs. We need experts in these jobs, not ex-policemen who lack credibility.' Indeed, the financial adviser responsible for developing the system and facilitating its implementation resigned and was not replaced for several years, consequently no one was 'batting' for the system within the organisation. So, it was hardly surprising that the introduction of the inspectors' financial accounting system was seriously delayed. Consequently, the police are still unable to make effective the crucial link between costs and outputs.

Work on developing activity measures started later – a joint Home Office/Inspectorate working group was not formed until 1986 – but progress has been more rapid. The intention was to construct a computerised set of indicators that would provide the other half of the costs/outputs equation. The premise was that although there were few obvious global indicators of police performance, the organisation was, in the words of one inspector, 'awash with statistics that had been around the forces for years but had never been systematically compiled and stored'; statistics that 'we might not have previously used to their full potential'. The result was the 'matrix of indicators': 'a computer-based system of key indicators to provide a guide to matters of efficiency in the principal functional areas of police activity'. The matrix transferred existing quantitative data into a computerised database compiled from forms annually submitted by each force to the Inspectorate.

The matrix consisted of 435 indicators allocated to various functional categories: organisational structure/manpower deployment and use, crime detection, criminal proceedings, traffic, recruitment and wastage, complaints, community relations/crime prevention/special constabulary, public order, drugs, and civilianisation. For example, there were forty-three indicators in the traffic category. These ranged from basic data about the number of officers dedicated to traffic duty, through details of incidents such as police vehicle accidents, breath tests, motoring offenders prosecuted, to indicators that touch on aspects of efficiency such as the number of breath tests per officer. The matrix allowed comparisons to be made over time, against a national average or with any other police force. However, no one claimed that these indicators were precise measures – in the words of one manager, many of the indicators were simply 'dressed-up data' – but they represented an important advance in the reliability and quality of activity and output information.

It is significant that the matrix was conceived, developed, and used by the Inspectorate when reviewing individual forces. The annual inspection is the basis for the allocation of the Home Office grant. The emphasis is firmly on peer review, illustrated in the words of a former chief inspector who declared that forces 'have nothing to fear from searching scrutinies by those who share your common aims and objectives for the police service, and whose professional judgement is based on wide practical knowledge and experience of the vicissitudes of policing' (Barratt 1986: 17). However, after 1983 the inspection became a more serious affair in which the inspectors helped set objectives, assessed their achievement, and had the new duty of examining 'financial information and control[ling] how costs are taken into account in considering the different options for deploying resources, and how value for money is ensured'. It is in this context that the Inspectorate was keen to improve the quality of information, simply to enable it to make some assessment of value for money.

The matrix was first used in 1986 to make comparisons between the ten or eleven forces covered by one individual inspector. Initially, unrealistic and unfair comparisons were made, for example between the large West Midlands force and the small Dyfed/Powys force; these did not prove very useful. Subsequently, more useful national comparisons across regions were possible between 'families' of forces with a similar sized establishment, or on urban/rural lines or various other demo-graphic and geographical dimensions (although time-series comparison was limited by the five-year limit to the matrix database). The original matrix was made inflexible by its dependence upon annually reported data; this is still largely true but some experiments have since been made with shorter time-spans, such as the monitoring of complaints on a three-monthly basis. A speedier system of monitoring was developed in key areas such as crime: enabling data to be obtained by the Inspectorate from forces within fourteen days so that all inter-force comparisons could be returned to individual forces for action within a month of the event reported. As a result the matrix has increasingly exposed forces to 'uncomfortable comparisons' (Joint Consultative Committee 1990).

Each of the five regional offices for the Inspectorate had computer access to the database facilitating the regular use of the matrix during inspections. The normal procedure was that about three weeks before an inspection, superintendents visit a force to examine the figures, ask preliminary and clarificatory questions, subsequently to follow-up the problems and issues that are uncovered. The matrix was then used to provide more detail on specific aspects of their findings, such as a comparison of the rates of absenteeism or of ethnic recruitment. Inspectors might take fifty indicators to an individual inspection, depending on the specific problems of a force. One inspector emphasised the importance of good presentation and communication: 'the information has to be presented in bar graphs that are immediately intelligible to the busy non-statistician – every picture must tell a story'. Thus the inspector might present a chief constable with a computerised bar graph comparing a specific indicator with others in that force's family showing simply and accurately how the performance of the individual force compares with the average. One example of its use involved a force that was very proud of its drugs record, yet the matrix showed that its drug squad had a worse record than others. The explanation was that officers were frequently pulled away from drugs duties whenever an emergency came up, so that in practice the high-profile drugs squad was proving ineffective.

The matrix of indicators is still under development but it is now referred to regularly in inspectors' reports and in their responses to requests for increases in establishment. Progress in implementing the matrix outstripped the financial system, although the latter had been set up some four years earlier. According to the Chief Inspector, the matrix:

> has become an indispensable tool at regional offices, as a supplement to HMIs professional judgement, and at Queen Anne's Gate [the Home Office] . . . progressively the results of analysis are being fed back to forces as part of the inspection process, when significant variations between broadly similar forces can be pursued . . . hoped [it] will encourage an increasingly productive dialogue on activity indicators and efficiency and effectiveness between the inspectorate and forces.
>
> (Chief Inspector of Constabulary 1989: 10)

It does seem that the inspectors have now accepted and use the matrix. Indeed, one or two inspectors are very enthusiastic about the way the matrix provides information across the spectrum of fiscal to operational matters:

> It provides us with a 'glimpse of the blindingly obvious'. We find it helps us to 'home in' on issues and to ask better and informed questions. It helps us to be altogether sharper in our work, considering the short time that we spend in any force during an inspection. We can be more analytical rather than just accepting the story we are told.

The improvement in question-asking was illustrated by the following tale:

> One force put a lot of effort into reducing car crime but their figures seemed no better than before. Using the matrix we found that the increase in recorded crime was largely due to the 'Beastie Boy' cult of stealing badges from Volkswagen cars. This crime was categorized alongside car thefts yet it is not what we would describe as a serious car crime, and probably one that cannot be resolved by police action. It was the matrix that allowed us to home in on it which we could not have done before.

The Inspectorate hopes to extend the use of the matrix from a simple question-asking technique into a 'persuasive tool' that will enable them to obtain greater influence over local forces. For example, a chief constable currently sets objectives with the advice of the inspector, who can then only assess a force on its own objectives. The matrix will allow the inspectors to point a chief constable towards a problem that needs resolving and so give a strong hint that it should form a force objective. Significantly, the matrix was actively promoted by the inspector who helped conceive it thus providing a lesson in organisational change by illustrating the advantages of having key personnel – product champions – with sufficient organisational status and commitment to win over doubters.

The inspectors were aware of the importance of 'selling it' to chief constables: 'there is an automatic resistance to any change. We must seep it into them until it becomes accepted as a way of life.' Nevertheless it appears that the matrix was received with little overt opposition, albeit with differing degrees of enthusiasm: 'there was no overt knocking of it . . . chief constables recognise that we are now better informed than they are about their own force and about trends – and this has helped us'. But, despite the enthusiasts, there are many chief constables who are privately dismissive of the matrix, seeing it as just one more burden to cope with. If there was genuine enthusiasm among chief constables then forces would surely be further ahead with computerisation so that they could utilise the matrix themselves. As one official ruefully commented: 'computerisation would at least help reduce the common complaint that there are too many forms to fill in and too much time being wasted providing information for 435 indicators!' Indeed, the Inspectorate may have fallen into the trap of generating too many 'indicators' thus inviting criticisms of unreliability, inflexibility, and time-wasting. It was a situation exacerbated by the existence of alternative, non-compatible information systems – the matrix, CIPFA statistics, Home Office returns, etc. – each collected and presented in different ways. There is clearly a need for a common police service information system with improved coverage, reliability, and less duplication (see also Joint Consultative Committee 1990).

A more significant criticism from within the service is that the Home Office and the Inspectorate are using the matrix as part of a broad strategy to bring in changes in operational methods and management culture. There is a widespread feeling, expressed clearly and intelligently by the Joint Consultative Committee (1990), that the pressure on the police from central and local government to increase productivity and display value for money has resulted in an excessive and undesirable interest in the 'measurable aspects of police work'. This trend can be seen in operational terms with the spread of techniques such as graded response and crime screening, and in managerial initiatives such as policing by objectives and the use of the matrix. It is widely held within the service that the focus on the quantifiable has occurred at the cost of the unquantifiable preventive and service functions that are essential ingredients of 'traditional' British policing. More specifically, critics point to the 'goal displacement' caused by the pursuit of measurable targets rather than essential objectives; a response that in its extreme manifestation led to the recent case of Kent officers who persuaded convicted prisoners to 'confess' to unsolved crimes for which they were innocent, thereby improving the clear-up rate of the individual officers. Such arguments, whatever their merits, illustrate the resistance of many chief constables to the wider use of PIs – whether it is due to fears for traditional policing and the dangers of goal displacement, the threat to the autonomy of the local force posed by the greater control that the matrix gives to the Home Office, or simply because chief constables are culture-bound and reluctant to change their ways. The fact that this opposition exists poses a major implementation problem for the Inspectorate and the Home Office.

This does not mean that forces have ignored PIs – the case of the Kent police officers mentioned above illustrates that PIs have exerted a significant influence – but that indicators are being used haphazardly, with little direction. When an inspector claims that 'the matrix is about changing the culture of the organisation' he needs to be sure that the new culture is better than the old. For example, how does the matrix fit in with the modern trend towards community policing when the whole object of community policing is to try to take people outside of the criminal justice system by not recording events and certain police activities. The matrix, by emphasising recorded data, appears to fly in the face of this approach.

The police has certainly become increasingly aware of the need to provide the service wanted by consumers; the problem being that the police serve so many constituencies, each with different and often contradictory wants and expectations from the service. Given these difficulties, it is questionable how useful consumer surveys are; nonetheless, in recent years several individual forces have commissioned surveys both of the public and of the force itself. Despite this concern, the amount of information about police performance that is available to the public is remarkably small. Given the importance that the Inspectorate seems to attach to the matrix, it is perhaps unfortunate that wider dissemination of the indicators has been limited to individual forces and, to a limited extent, via the chief constable, to police authorities.

The complex nature of accountability within the police is reflected in its performance indicators. Just as police accountability has been described as 'a Babel of evaluative languages with little agreement about which should be used and by whom where' (Day and Klein 1987: 105), so the conflicting reasons, responsibility, and enthusiasm for developing PIs has meant that progress has been slow, confused, and widely resisted. The police coped with the pressure to respond to the FMI without generating hostility from below by allotting primary responsibility for the development of PIs to the Inspectorate and thereby containing the reforms within existing structures of performance review. Thus the matrix was designed as an instrument with which the Inspectorate could exercise better 'hands-off' control over individual forces.

The police, like the NHS, has to wrestle with some of the most intractable problems of performance assessment facing any of our services and there have been no startling developments in the measurements of efficiency, effectiveness, or, least of all, quality. Not surprisingly, the focus of the matrix, and similar initiatives at force level, is on intermediate outputs and activities. Nonetheless, despite the limitations of this highly data-driven system, the Inspectorate and the Home Office are clearly able to exercise greater control over individual forces because they now possess detailed information about police activity. Moreover, as these computerised systems become more widely available at force level so chief constables will be able to exercise greater control over their own organisation.

The matrix is, however, a rather crude set of indicators. The continuing pressure to develop better PIs, expressed in a speech to the Police Foundation in 1988 by the Home Secretary and underlined in Home Office Circular 35/1989, seems to be greater than at the time circular 114/1983 was published. Given the poor response of individual forces to that circular and its exhortation to construct PIs, the Joint Consultative Committee believes that the Home Office 'will impose a wide range of common performance indicators, which the service has had little or no influence in developing'. The Home Office quite clearly intends that those PIs will provide one further means of increasing central control over the police service.

THE LORD CHANCELLOR'S DEPARTMENT

The court service of the Lord Chancellor's Department (LCD) has the lowest profile of the three core parts of the criminal justice system covered in this chapter, but the need to allow for the whims of idiosyncratic judges and others in the legal profession ensures that the assessment of organisational performance is an often hazardous process. Indeed, although part of the criminal justice system, as an organisation seeking to assess its performance, the LCD has more in common with our welfare deliverers: Social Security and the NHS. The aims of the LCD range from the provision of access to justice, to the safeguard of judicial appointments, but this chapter is concerned with its primary aim of providing a fast, efficient, and cost-effective court system.

The work of the LCD consists of criminal business (44 per cent of expenditure in 1988–9), civil business (49 per cent), and court building (7 per cent). Criminal work is disposed of by the Crown Court and civil work by the County Courts, with the support of various higher and lower courts such as the Court of Appeal. The department is organised into six regional circuits each controlled by a Circuit Administrator. Within each circuit there are a number of areas each managed by a Courts Administrator under whom is a Chief Clerk responsible for individual local offices. This conventional hierarchical management structure is responsible for the administration of approximately 400 courts and some 600 premises, although the size of individual offices can vary between two and 120 staff.

The Lord Chancellor's Department is entirely within the public sector. The Crown Courts are a non-trading business but in civil proceedings the gross costs of running the County Courts are largely offset by fees charged for the services provided by the department. Consequently, while the Crown Courts obviously provide a monopoly service, a competitive element exists in the County Courts because their use is influenced by the potential costs of the legal process; a litigant may choose not to carry through a case or seek to settle 'out of court' in order to reduce costs. As a central government department, the LCD is directly accountable to Parliament. However, the LCD does not have a particularly high political profile: not surprisingly parliamentary and media attention tends to focus on controversial sentencing decisions by the judiciary (over which the department exercises no jurisdiction) rather than the administration of the court system. The work of the LCD is relatively homogeneous; essentially it is concerned with administering the quick, efficient passage of caseloads through the judicial system (with no concern for the outcome of the case); in this respect it is similar to Social Security, our other caseload department, which is responsible for the fast, accurate payment of welfare benefits. Likewise, it is also low on uncertainty. As long as every facility is provided to enable a fair hearing to take place within a reasonable period of time, then the department can be fairly sure that it is achieving its aim; the relationship between throughput and outcome is relatively straightforward.

However, in contrast with Social Security, and more in common with the NHS, the Lord Chancellor's Department is quite high on complexity. The task of the court listings officer – the key individual charged with planning the schedules of trials – is complicated by particular problems of performance ownership arising from the need to work interdependently with the judiciary, the legal profession, and their clients. Thus the speed with which cases are brought to trial hinges on the interdependent actions and tactics of the various groups of barristers and solicitors concerned with a particular case. Once started, the length of a trial can vary enormously. The work rate of the judge – like that of a doctor – albeit under some constraint to work a minimum length day, varies widely between individuals. More important, as a not-guilty plea necessitates a full trial, so the lower the 'plea rate' (i.e. the higher the number of not-guilty pleas) the greater the court time taken up, hence the slower the throughput of cases. The listings officer, like the hospital manager, therefore confronts a serious problem of case-mix: just as there is a significant variation in the time needed for different operations (and differences between individuals), so some types of case take much longer to complete than others: a complex murder trial may span several weeks or months whilst several 'petty' burglaries can be cleared up in a morning. The court listings officer tries to take these factors into account when planning the schedule of hearings, but because so many of these factors are beyond her or his control, or require careful planning and negotiation, the officer can at best only estimate the length of time that a case will take. In short, the department faces a significant problem of performance ownership.

The design and use of performance indicators in the Lord Chancellor's Department

There is little evidence to suggest that the department attributed much importance to performance evaluation prior to 1979. There was a long history of measuring basic activities, such as the disposal rate of committals and cases and the length of time that defendants have to wait before their case comes to trial. However, these data were used primarily for the official recording of trends (published in the annual *Judicial Statistics*), rather than the evaluation of organisational performance. The change of government in 1979 had little immediate impact; the only notable result of the Rayner era was a marginal reform of costing systems. Nevertheless in the new era of resource constraint the department recognised that a system of priority setting was necessary, particularly in the light of the increase in workload. There was a massive increase of 46 per cent in Crown Court committals during the period 1982–7 and a rise of 3 per cent per annum in civil court business since 1980 (HM Treasury 1988). Thus the seeds of organisational change were sown, but senior managers acknowledged that the FMI was, as one put it, the 'trigger' for reform. The main thrust of the initial response to the FMI focused on setting up a management accounting system that brought together running costs, staffing, and receipts to allow quick and accurate costings of court operations in their functional activities. The system was based on some 400 cost centres located in local court offices. These units were also to be the basis of the future budgetary delegation which, thus far, has reached the level of the Court Administrator. By the end of the 1980s, Circuit Administrators were setting financial performance targets for the Court Administrator.

Some progress was also made towards improving performance measurement although the department was, as one manager put it, 'travelling from a low starting point'. One public sign of a new interest was a brief reference in the Public Expenditure White Paper in 1983 to average waiting times for defendants facing trial. But the introduction of *Circuit Objectives* in 1984 represented the first serious attempt to translate the wealth of statistics into a set of internal performance-related targets. These objectives were initially rather crude and narrow in their coverage. However, following the recommendations of an internal working party set up to evaluate the first two years' use of circuit objectives, the sophistication and coverage of the circuit objectives were improved.

The circuit objectives were developed first in the Crown Courts, for both political and technical reasons. The Crown Courts deal with what staff call 'liberty of the individual' issues which tend to receive most political limelight; in particular the department is under constant pressure to reduce the time that defendants have to wait in custody prior to their trial. Further pressure came from the Treasury which was particularly concerned about the efficiency of the Crown Courts because they are funded almost entirely from the government coffers (unlike the civil courts which are largely fee-paying). Technically, more data about Crown Court activities existed because, as we shall see, it is simply harder to devise measures of civil court performance. The following analysis of the development of these circuit objectives adopts the distinction between the Crown and civil courts.

The main activity of the LCD is the disposal of cases. This is most apparent in the Crown Courts where the trial is the focus of the circuit objectives: the trial has a clear beginning and end which makes it a convenient unit of measurement. When the department constructed its PIs the data recording the 'waiting time' for the committal of a case for trial were already available, so it was a relatively simple matter to transform these data into performance indicators by calculating the percentage of defendants whose cases had not reached court by a certain time period. The first circuit objectives set annual targets for each circuit measuring the 'percentage of committals for trial outstanding' for three benchmark periods of eight, thirteen, and thirty-six weeks. These objectives were disaggregated both geographically by region and by distinguishing defendants in custody and on bail. Subsequent adjustments to the system meant that the circuit objectives targeted the average waiting time for all defendants rather than the percentage still waiting after a specified period (see Table 3.2). For example, in line with political priorities the Lord Chancellor was keen that all circuits, with the exception of South Eastern which has a far heavier caseload, should be targeted to achieve an average waiting time for custody cases of eight weeks.

In addition to the key committal waiting time objective, there were a number of circuit objectives targeting the waiting time for sentencing and for disposing of appeals (the percentage of defendants or appellants

Table 3.2 Crown Court: committals for trial – average waiting time (in weeks) of defendants dealt with 1983–4 to 1988–9 (England and Wales)

	1983–4	1984–5	1985–6	1986–7	1987–8	1988–9
Defendants in custody	9.8	10.1	10.2	10.3	9.8	10.1
Defendants on bail	15.4	15.3	15.2	14.9	12.6	13.3
All defendants	14.3	14.2	14.0	13.9	12.0	12.5

Source: HM Treasury (1990), Cmnd. 1009

Table 3.3 Crown Court: average hours sat per day 1984–5 to 1988–9 (England and Wales)

	1984–5	1985–6	1986–7	1987–8	1988–9
Average hours sat per day	4.9	5.0	5.2	5.0	4.2*

* Excludes lunch hour following change in definition in April 1988
Source: HM Treasury 1990, Cmnd. 1009

still waiting after four weeks). Another circuit objective set a target for determination (the time that bills to solicitors and counsel remain unpaid). All the PIs discussed so far are throughput measures that represent a reasonably valid proxy for effectiveness; in short, if the speed with which the departmental caseload is processed can be increased then, assuming quality is held constant, this implies a more effective achievement of objectives.

Efficiency has proven a harder nut to crack. One way of improving the use of resources is to increase the length of the 'sitting day' – the average hours in which the court is in session each day (see Table 3.3). Unlike the other circuit objectives, this was an indicator which the department wanted to see *increase* – and it has had some success in recent years. A second efficiency objective, introduced in 1988, measured the use of jurors. Payments to jurors represent about one sixth of the total expenditure on criminal business (including judicial costs but excluding the costs of legal representation), hence it is an enormous waste of resources to summon jurors who then are not used to sit in a trial. So the new PI recorded the percentage of juror non-sitting days against attendance days. However, as this was a completely new measure, the department found it hard to assess the level at which this PI should be targeted. After an initial trial period it was decided to set each circuit the objective of ensuring that all jurors were sitting for at least 70 per cent of the days when they attend court.

There were also some PIs measuring Crown Court efficiency that were not yet part of the circuit objective system because they were still being monitored and evaluated. These were unit costings: running cost per disposal, running cost per court room day, and disposals per member of staff. They provide reasonable proxies for some areas of court work but central managers recognised that they are not comprehensive and, because 'so many factors are outside our control', it is possible that 'quite dangerous' interpretations could be drawn from these figures. In particular, one manager observed that 'the PIs assume that Crown Court units are comparable but they aren't: plea rates, the length of cases all vary across and between circuits'. Nevertheless, in the LCD as in other organisations, managers were generally grateful for the descriptive indicator simply because of its capacity to pose questions without giving definitive answers: 'for example, a high plea rate would lead us to expect a low cost per disposal: now at least we can look at the figures to see if this is true'.

The performance of the civil courts is more difficult to measure than that of the Crown Courts because the role of the trial is less central: many cases never reach court, there is no single unit of measurement and, consequently, activity data are less comprehensive. Managers describe the civil courts as 'paper factories': the broad aim is to 'improve the throughput of cases from initial application and at every stage leading to resolution of disputes and enforcement of judgments and orders' (HM Treasury 1988). Consequently, the civil court circuit objectives focused on the time taken to complete various items of process. When first introduced the circuit objectives measured the percentage of courts on a circuit where five key items of process – originating process, enforcement process, Judge's and Registrar's Orders, entry of judgment, and divorce petitions – were left outstanding after five days. However, because it was the larger courts that tended to miss targets this meant that the 'true' performance was 'somewhat concealed by the way of measuring it', resulting in misleading figures. Subsequently, the department measured what it called the 'volume of process' for the same five major areas of 'staff-led work' (see Table 3.4).

These PIs are still less satisfactory than the Crown Court measures. Central managers acknowledged this problem:

> We know that this system does not capture the full breadth of activity but we would say that there is no need to do so and it would create too much work for staff to try to be comprehensive. Yet the staff use this as a criticism of the system; they complain, for example, that we don't look at the time taken to deal with correspondence.

Table 3.4 County Court: the percentage of processes taking longer than five days to issue and dispatch

	1987–8	1988–9
Original process	31.2	10.6
Enforcement process	30.4	15.5
Entry of judgment	23.2	12.9
Divorce petitions	17.8	7.5
Orders	44.2	30.1

Source: HM Treasury 1990, Cmnd. 1009

These objections notwithstanding, the department imposed a standardised required performance across the country on all five items and, like the Crown Court, on the length of judge's sitting day. These targets were not open to negotiation by the individual circuits: as a result 'we can now ask questions why specific areas cannot perform to these standards'.

Two further throughput objectives targeted the percentage of courts where the waiting time for a registrar's hearing is more than six weeks and for a judge's hearing more than eight weeks, but there were no standardised targets for this PI. As with the Crown Courts a further objective was to increase the average hours of court usage per sitting day, just like, as we shall see, hospital managers trying to intensify the use of operating theatres. More recently a new PI was introduced extending the circuit objective system to the work of bailiffs. There was a 'success target' that was intended to minimise the percentage of warrants where payment has not been secured, and a throughput target that aimed to reduce the number of warrants in the system that are over one month old. The weakness of these two PIs is that they assess the speed and success of a process that is not really within the control of bailiffs. Moreover, as managers acknowledged, 'on the one hand, the plaintiffs want the money but, on the other hand, the bailiff cannot chase it up every week'; in other words, the bailiff must be given sufficient latitude to balance the often conflicting concerns of speed, efficiency, and success.

The department has found it difficult to develop robust efficiency PIs for the civil courts. The existing efficiency PIs were based on the notion of unit values: namely, 'cost per unit' which measured staff costs plus overheads (excluding judicial and accommodation costs). Unit costings are more useful in the civil courts than in the Crown Courts because there is a direct correlation between staff and work. However, there is some dissatisfaction with this measure because it 'gives an idea of workload but not complexity'; in other words it does not allow for the eternal problem of case-mix. Furthermore, the absence of identifiable output measures (currently only throughput measures are used) and hence the capacity to accumulate costs for that output undermine the validity of unit cost efficiency measures. However, the department is under constant pressure from the Treasury to continue 'improving and looking for efficiency measures and it is required to produce evidence of an increase in productivity'; to this end it has set a national target for an increase in workload of 2.5 per cent a year between 1990 and 1991 and 1992 and 1993 (HM Treasury 1990).

Since the introduction of the circuit objectives system the basic approach has remained the same, but there has been a constant process of monitoring and evaluation which, in turn, produced improvements in the methods of data collection, the marginal alteration of certain objectives, and, as we have seen, the extension of the system to previously uncovered areas of work. Thus, for example, considerable efforts were directed at improving the data upon which the circuit objectives were based so that the reliability of the PIs has improved. For instance, annual performance was initially measured solely on 31 March each year which provided a static snapshot of performance capable of distortion by an abnormal event, such as a water authority issuing all its credit work the day before; this system has been replaced by a cumulative form of measurement.

Apart from getting the techniques right, there has also been a gradual integration of the target-setting process into the system of management. PIs have become an accepted tool of management that, in particular, have strengthened the relationship between performance and resource allocation. The circuit objectives were integrated into the management process as a top-down system of target-setting, stretching down from Deputy-Secretary to line manager. Initially, the key event was the annual bilateral negotiation between the Deputy-Secretary and the six Circuit Administrators that set circuit performance targets based on the results from the previous year, the anticipated workload, and the available resources. These targets were 'intended to represent a level of performance that is testing yet realistic in the circumstances of the circuit' (NAO 1986: 49). The targets were quite 'crude' in 1985, the first year of its operation, but subsequently they improved as, on the one hand, headquarters became more probing and, on the other hand, circuit administrators were better prepared to defend targets and performance. However, the department became increasingly confident about its ability to set precise, realistic targets so that by the late 1980s it had largely dispensed with the system of negotiated targets: 'there is now a standardised required performance across the country on the five major Crown Court items and on the length of the sitting day; these targets are now imposed on the circuits, not negotiated'. Presumably as the teething troubles of bailiffs and jurors' objectives are ironed out so they too will be imposed on the circuits.

Each circuit administrator disaggregates this standard target into targets for individual courts. Some circuits simply adopt the average circuit figure across every court; others calculate targets for each individual court making allowance for specific circumstances such as staffing, workload, and location (NAO 1986: 49). As the centre sees only the aggregated circuit statistics rather than a breakdown of individual court performance, headquarters is content to leave the strategy for achieving targets to the discretion of circuit administrators: 'we would not dictate to a Court Administrator; that is up the Circuit Administrator'. On the one hand, the individually tailored approach encourages greater involvement and support from staff who applaud the attempt to capture the unique circumstances of each office but, on the other hand, it makes larger demands on resources.

The performance data are collated weekly in local offices, passed monthly to region, and quarterly to headquarters. Planned and actual performance against the circuit objectives was initially assessed at national level annually, then biannually, but latterly the centre has carried out a quarterly review: 'We now have a more comprehensive package of PIs and we can operate more quickly. With experience we can ask better questions about the figures that allow us to focus on under-achievers.'

The Circuit Administrator attempts to enlist all staff into the collective pursuit of circuit objectives:

> I have to secure realistic targets from the 'Grade Two' and ensure that these are achieved by the 'troops', so I need to constantly review them. The Courts Administrator will take decisions about redeploying resources and resolving issues but if problems persist then I must determine whether it is a resource or personnel problem. I must explain why performance differs from targets . . . The purpose of PIs is as a management tool – it is making people aware that we have objectives to achieve – so although the system needs refinement it is a good base for concentrating the minds of clerks.

At each level managers expect to receive 'an explanation for a shortfall' but there are no explicit sanctions for a failure to achieve targets. The monthly circulation of Crown Court figures to the region seems to have encouraged the development of 'a strong circuit loyalty'. Indeed, there is even frequent reference to the informal 'league tables' that compare the performance of the different circuits: 'Ten years ago the existence of a league table would have produced a strike but now everyone is absolutely frantic to get hold of one!' These league tables are produced in response to a bottom-up demand ('it is the Circuit Administrator who provides them, not headquarters'); the change in philosophy being well illustrated by the tendency for circuit administrators to discuss the league tables with their counterparts, whereas previously it was a subject that was never spoken about.

Significantly one Deputy-Secretary has been made responsible for both the allocation of resources and the setting of targets. This is regarded as an important intellectual link within the department but it is a link that requires considerable improvement: 'the relationship between resources and objectives is not straightforward and it is unlikely ever to be mathematically measurable because there will always be some intuition involved'. In other words, it is very difficult to integrate the resources and objectives when workload, disposal rates, and available court days are, as we have seen, subject to such wide and often unpredictable fluctuations. Nevertheless, signs of improvement were noted by the National Audit Office (1986: 49) during the first years of the circuit objectives system, and within the department it is held that 'the circuits are more conscious now of what they have to do', performance figures are increasingly incorporated into the budgetary process and there is frequent talk about a 'contract to perform' so that 'for "x" money we should produce "y" performance'.

Nevertheless there are a number of problems with the circuit objectives system that the department has not yet overcome. First, as those responsible for designing and implementing the system see it, the lack of a satisfactory input/output ratio makes any calculation of efficiency very difficult. So, for example, despite the recent introduction of new efficiency measures it is still difficult to provide a confident answer to a basic question such as whether the steady reduction in overall Crown Court average waiting times in recent years represents improved efficiency when set against, on the one hand, an increase in workload of 46 per cent over the same period or, on the other hand, the benefits of a larger allocation of resources.

Second, because the Lord Chancellor's Department is a 'caseload' department the use of throughput indicators does represent a reasonable proxy for effectiveness: for example, as we have seen, waiting time is a good indicator of Crown Court effectiveness because the main task of the department is to get cases to trial as quickly as possible. However, the indicators of average waiting time are unsophisticated; in particular, they fail to take into account three of the key variables discussed above: the plea-rate, the case-mix, and judicial behaviour. For example, the Crown Courts are commonly described as 'judge-driven': the court listings officer has little control over the length of the judges' day and the personal idiosyncrasies of a judge. Circuit objectives are made available to judges but, apart from encouraging judges to minimise the number of adjournments, managers would 'not presume' to ask a judge to speed up; just as the consultant exercises complete professional autonomy within the operating theatre, so the judge presides unchallenged in the courtroom. The court listings officer tries to take these independent factors into account, but a great deal of unpredictability remains. Indeed, the observation is frequently made within the service that the circuit objectives only really measure the skill of individual listings officers: clearly some means of building these uncontrollable factors into the objective setting system would considerably improve the quality of target-setting, but it is not obvious how this could be achieved.

Third, several of the circuit objectives fail to take account of the impact that variations in court size can have on performance. For example, the imposition of a standard target for the number of days that a juror must sit when in attendance at court may impose an unfairly onerous burden on a small court: whilst a large court can find places within its own set-up for those jurors who are not needed, a small, geographically remote court may be prevented from redeployment to neighbouring courts by virtue of the long distances involved.

Fourth, there are no quality indicators other than waiting time. The department is concerned about the possible conflict between speed and quality. One solution is to obtain some measure of the number and type of complaints. The problem is that complaints rarely relate to the *administration* of the service but to the way in which a case was handled by the judge, or about the actual judgment; factors that are beyond the control of the department. Nor is there any consumer input to the target-setting process to help determine what is acceptable performance. One difficulty is to decide who the consumers are and whether their preferences coincide with those of the department. We can use the example of the departmental objective of reducing the waiting time of defendants remanded in custody. Thus, if the consumer is the taxpayer concerned about costs, or the innocent defendant who is deprived of his or her freedom, then the department would presumably find support for its policy. But if the consumer is the *guilty* defendant then they might prefer to wait as long as possible in custody because the conditions on remand are better than those facing a convicted prison inmate!

Lastly, as in many other departments the sudden pressure following the introduction of the FMI meant that the circuit objectives system was fitted to existing available data. This has proven less of a problem than in organisations such as the NHS, but the court data were clearly better suited to the evaluation of effectiveness than of efficiency. More generally, the system still depends on rather 'primitive' manual recording systems.

Despite these problems, managers at the centre believe that there has generally been a 'pretty good reaction' to the circuit objectives. There was some initial suspicion about the system: regional management saw it as an attempt by the centre to reduce their traditional autonomy; middle and junior management believed it was a tool for introducing a cut in resources; and there was a widespread fear among staff that the circuit objectives would lead to reductions in staffing levels, or to increased workloads. Most of this resistance has now been overcome, but the department, like others, may need to work at improving bottom-up involvement in the production and achievement of circuit objectives because, as the NAO report found, some Chief Clerks in charge of individual courts considered the targets to be unrealistic. Moreover, as long as the PIs are unable to distinguish adequately between factors that depend on the performance of staff and those that are externally driven, there will remain a degree of reserve and even hostility to the system. This said, as one senior manager observed, opposition to the system dissipated when managers realised that the circuit objectives can be used 'in their favour; i.e. to prove that they have a heavy workload and need extra resources!'

The introduction of the circuit objectives system in the Lord Chancellor's Department represented a relatively successful response to the pressure generated by the FMI to improve performance measurement. It was a data-driven system that, at least in the case of the Crown Courts division, benefited from the existence of the trial as an easily measurable and definable yardstick for assessing performance. The absence of conflict over objectives and the narrow focus of performance ensured a rare parsimony in the number of PIs produced: a few key indicators provide a fairly comprehensive and uncontroversial coverage of departmental activity. Thus it was possible for the circuit objectives to be fairly well integrated into the planning and budgeting processes, overcoming the usual organisational resistance with less difficulty than other departments.

A critical factor in the successful implementation of the circuit objectives was the constant process of monitoring, reforming, and extending the system. As an interim measure it was possible to introduce crude data-driven circuit objectives but subsequently many weaknesses have been ironed out. Staff may still complain, often with good reason, that performance against targets depends to a significant degree on factors that are beyond the control of managers, but it seems fair to say that the system has been largely accepted and is being used throughout the service.

THE PRISON SERVICE

Of all the organisations studied in this book the prison service has been traditionally the most secretive about its performance; the locked doors symbolise not just its function but also the view of its members as isolated from the community. Thus, despite not being a professional group, prison officers have managed to minimise external scrutiny of their performance and are therefore probably the most invisible workforce of all our organisations. Indeed, perhaps more than in any other organisation, the recent interest in performance monitoring can be seen as one part of a broader management strategy to bring the workforce under control. Progress implementing the FMI has been slow, but the prison service has produced a performance measurement system that is in important respects quite different from those found in most other public sector services; a feature that is partly explained by organisational characteristics that distinguish the prison system from other services.

The responsibility for holding prisoners in custody resides entirely within the public sector. Prisons provide a non-trading service, except for the token proceeds arising from the sale of produce generated by the labour of prisoners. The prison service in England and Wales has a virtual monopoly over the custody of prisoners (although there are always a number of inmates held in police cells): in 1989–90 an estimated 32,800 staff looked after 49,800 inmates in 125 establishments (HM Treasury 1990: Cmnd. 1009). Although management does not have to contend with any significant professional groups, the prison officers are, as has already been noted, one of the most powerful and well-organised occupational groupings in the public sector; consequently, management is a process of negotiation and consent rather than dictat and coercion. One sign of the power of the prison officers is that there are almost as many gaolers as prisoners. The Prison Department administers four regions each incorporating a number of penal establishments. The four regional directors control and are accountable for the performance of each establishment within their region. In practice, the regional directors and prison governors enjoy a considerable degree of autonomy, but the existence of direct lines of authority enables the Home Office to exercise 'hands on' control when necessary, as it did during the Strangeways riot in 1990 when the prison governor was prevented from ordering his officers to storm immediately the buildings 'occupied' by inmates. This example also illustrates the extent to which prisons are in the public eye; when things go wrong in prisons they feel the weight of ministerial pressure more quickly than almost any other organisation.

The prison service ranks middle to low on heterogeneity and low on complexity. Although the basic custodial function of the service implies homogeneity of task, in each establishment there may also be accommodation units, educational and training facilities, workshops, catering, and possibly a hospital complex, all of which require different staff, skills, and resources. The performance of these various functions is generally quite autonomous and does not therefore require a complex set of interdependent tasks.

The dimension of uncertainty is less straightforward. First, there is uncertainty over organisational objectives. On the one hand, the primary aim of prisons – the secure custody of inmates – poses few conceptual problems: the objective is quite simply to stop anyone escaping by running an establishment that minimises the opportunities to abscond. On the other hand, the prison service is also expected to pursue additional aims, such as the reformation and rehabilitation of inmates. These objectives may conflict: can a penal system geared towards secure custody seriously attempt the rehabilitation of inmates through education and training? Second, there is uncertainty regarding the tenuous relationship between those objectives and any measurable outcomes. Whilst it is easy to judge the success of the custodial function by simply counting the number of escapes, it is quite hard to translate broad aims of rehabilitation into specific objectives against which performance can be measured.

To take one example, it has long been debated within the criminology literature whether it is within the power of the prison service somehow to 're-educate' inmates so that they are less likely to commit crimes again after their release. Certainly the organisation comes replete with educationalists, psychologists, and the provision of various opportunities for inmates to learn useful skills that may help secure employment after their release (on the questionable assumption that a successful incorporation into stable economic activity will reduce the motive to commit crime). But can a closed regime provide a suitable arena for change? Perhaps the style of regime matters more? On the one hand, it could be argued that the more unpleasant the experience of prison the less likely it is that an individual will risk returning; on the other hand, the unpleasant, cramped conditions which put criminals in close proximity to each other may simply magnify the likelihood of returning to a 'life of crime' (at the risk of being mechanistic, this could be compared to the dangers of cross-infection in hospitals). But it may be that the experience of prison has very little effect on criminal motivation; rather a whole series of environmental and personal factors, such as the level of unemployment or individual circumstances, may combine to influence the level of recidivism (Clarke and Cornish 1983; Goldman 1984). In this respect, prisons may not own their performance.

Thus, if we regard the prison service as simply concerned with the custodial function, then it is a straightforward task to set objectives and measure performance. If, as it has to be, the prison service is expected to satisfy various broad, humanitarian aims, then the task of performance measurement is more uncertain. If we accept that the prison service is concerned with something more than just the custodial function, then it differs markedly from both the Lord Chancellor's Department and the police. Unlike the courts, prisons do not have a caseload with a clear, definable throughput, and nor do its managers have to negotiate a complex set of interdependent work relationships. Unlike the police, the prison service has clear lines of accountability, provides a less heterogeneous service, and is not burdened by such a broad range of objectives.

The design and use of performance indicators in the prison service

The prison service has long displayed a reluctance to construct reliable information systems or to develop sophisticated performance measures. Apart from measuring the number of escapes, the one consistent attempt to assess prison effectiveness has been to measure the number of reconvictions as a means of evaluating the level of recidivism among former inmates. The problems of this indicator have already been noted. Prison managers have eschewed PIs, preferring what critics have described as a 'fire-fighting' approach, whereby they have often only become aware of poor performance as operations break down and, in extreme cases, the tiles come raining down on the heads of prison officers. Nor, until recently, has the prison service come under strong political pressure to account for its performance. Like the police, the prison system benefited from the commitment of the Thatcher Government to expand the law and order functions: the prison budget grew substantially in absolute terms and as a percentage of GDP during the 1980s, the department avoided the brunt of the initial attack on civil service 'inefficiency', and, subsequently, it was able to adopt a rather leisurely response to the FMI.

However, in recent years the Government has become increasingly concerned by the inadequacy of management costing systems and by the lack of PIs. To some extent the change in government attitude during the mid- to late-1980s was prompted by the publicity given to one negative PI – the 'roofs-off' indicator as it is called within the service – namely the sight of prisoners on the roof flashed across the news headlines; there can be few better examples of an alarm-bell PI that generates an immediate apoplectic response amongst Home Office Ministers. But government concern about prison performance had deeper roots.

The May Committee of Inquiry (Home Office 1979) had drawn attention to several internal organisational problems in the prison department. One recommendation involved 'opening up' the prison service to greater public scrutiny, hence its recommendation, accepted by the Home Secretary in 1980, to set up an external inspectorate (though based in the Home Office). The Chief Inspector's 'charter' required the inspection programme to focus on 'the morale of staff and prisoners; the quality of the regime; the conditions of buildings; questions of humanity and propriety; and the extent to which the establishment is giving value for money' (quoted in Morgan 1985: 110). In stating that its eventual aim was 'to establish benchmarks which will enable inspectors to assess establishments more objectively and with greater consistency' (quoted in Dunbar 1985: 74) it was recognised that there was insufficient information available for the inspectorate to carry out its role effectively.

A brief survey of published records illustrates the paucity of good quality information. Basic custodial data are published in *Prison Statistics*: these consist mostly of straightforward population statistics but the figures for the number of escapes disaggregated to the level of the individual prison (or regime as it is known in the trade) allows the organisation to evaluate the successful achievement of its basic aim. Additional data record the number of punishments meted out to unruly inmates for offences such as assaults on officers or fellow inmates, disobedience, and idleness. The usefulness of these measures is uncertain; although disaggregated to regime level they may represent negative indicators warning regional directors of underlying problems in individual institutions. Several measures of recidivism are also published. The Public Expenditure White Paper still includes no more than a few token indicators. There is one efficiency PI – the annual 'real operating cost per inmate' (£14,011 in 1988–9) – and a productivity measure – 'the number of inmate hours (hours in custody) per hour worked by officers' (11.1 hours in 1988–9) – but these are of limited use because they cannot be disaggregated to establishment level (HM Treasury 1990: Cmnd. 1009).

The primitive nature of prison information systems was underlined in an important internal report *A Sense of Direction*: 'it was not possible to know what was happening either in the system as a whole, or in different establishments, other than by impressionistic and incomplete sets of information required from time to time, as public interest or the need to know dictated' (Dunbar 1985: 48). Thus, for example, it had proven impossible to provide the May Committee with the cost data for individual establishments. Nor did the situation improve significantly for most of the 1980s. The newly formed inspectorate admitted that the poor availability of data had continued to impair its work (Morgan 1985) and the National Audit Office (1986) noted that informational flaws were particularly acute for the construction of PIs: 'progress in developing (these) output measures was slow because the necessary data was either unreliable or lacking' (43).

In view of these organisational weaknesses, it is hardly surprising that the Government began to look with despair at the performance of the prison service:

> Between 1978/79 and 1985/86 the number of prison officers increased by nearly 19 per cent, while the average inmate population rose by less than 12 per cent. Over the same period expenditure on the prison service rose by 36 per cent in real terms.
>
> (*Public Money* 1987, December: 57)

Put simply, where were the results of the enormous government commitment to the prison service? The apparent inefficiency highlighted by these figures was substantiated in an internal report by management consultants (ibid.).

The Prison Department responded to growing ministerial pressure to improve efficiency in a number of ways. The controversial 'Fresh Start' agreement negotiated with the Prison Officers Association has received most publicity: this scheme introduced flexible working arrangements aimed at reducing the working week to thirty-nine hours by 1992 thereby radically reducing the enormous amount of overtime worked by prison staff. But the department has also improved the way prison costings are collated and monitored. In response to the FMI it encouraged a move to devolved budgets: each regime now exercises considerable control over its own budget. The 'Prison Costing System' divided the functions of a regime into thirty cost centres which were related to activities. The cost centre functions were introduced in 1983/4 but the data were not published until 1987 because of worries about their accuracy. Indeed, the Prison Department still lacks accurate information about the allocation of staff time to particular activities. Although the centre has mooted a wide range of possible cost indicators – cost per inmate hour locked and unlocked, cost per visit, cost of a meal – it proved impossible accurately to cost functions from the centre without better staff time and cost data. Clearly, if inputs and outputs were ever to be properly linked, it was essential to have a system for monitoring prison activities.

The first step towards resolving this problem came from the Home Office. The May Committee had found that the existence of widespread confusion within the prison service over its aims and tasks was critical in explaining the manifold weaknesses in prison management systems (see also King and Morgan 1980). This uncertainty – whether the aims of the prison service should be humane containment, rehabilitation, or, in the words of the May Committee, 'positive custody' – has already been discussed; the point here is that this uncertainty was increasingly seen as a problem within the service.

One attempted solution was the 'Accountable Regimes' experiment which encouraged the setting of realistic local regime objectives (Chaplin 1982; Marsden and Evans 1985). Subsequently, this was superseded by the need to respond to the FMI with its exhortation to construct explicit objectives for the purpose of assessing performance. This prompted the Prison Board to formulate a 'Statement of the Tasks of the Prison Service', published as an appendix to Home Office circular 55/1984 (1984; see also Train 1985). The document emphasised the importance of using resources with 'maximum efficiency' in pursuit of the objectives of remand, security, humane treatment, and the preparation of prisoners for release, and it outlined a general framework for reviewing the work of the department at a strategic level. The accompanying 'Statement of the Functions of Prison Department Establishments' provided the means for regional directors and governors to 'discharge a similar responsibility in relation to individual establishments'. Christopher Train, Director General of the prison service, described these documents as representing an 'essentially pragmatic' approach, which 'does not include "aspirational" language' (Train 1985: 182). Put differently, Dunbar (1985) observed that the documents concentrate on the question 'What are we doing?' rather than 'Why are we here?'; by shifting the focus to functions rather than aims, it became more accessible to practitioners. Crucially, the documents provided the launching pad for the development of PIs by isolating factors over which the prison service could claim some ownership.

The initiative for the new management information system came from the *regional* level where managers had become increasingly concerned that their information systems gave them little idea of what actually happens inside a prison: for example, the number of punishments meted out to inmates indicates when things are going wrong, but what are regimes doing the rest of the time? In short, there was very little information about the activities and outputs of regimes. The publication of Circular 55/1984 by the Home Office was significant because it insisted that a 'functions document' for each establishment be negotiated between the regional director and the governor. This contract defined the functions of the individual establishment in the light of the broad criteria set out in the circular and in the context of specific local needs and available resources. In addition, there was a linked process whereby planned levels of performance, or 'baselines' (not minimum standards), were agreed. These baselines were expressed in terms of 'planned levels of the operating hours and the number of inmates involved in regime activities such as education, industries, other work parties and physical education' (Evans 1987: 10). The innovatory element of the functions document was that it provided the basis for assessing actual performance against planned performance. Previously, what was lacking was the information necessary to make such an evaluation: now, this 'missing link' could be replaced by a complete revision of the monitoring systems.

If the functions document provided a way into the puzzle the second part of the solution consisted of a new governor's 'weekly monitoring system' which was introduced in all four regions during 1987–8. The system had three stated purposes: to monitor effective service delivery; to assist management control by prompting informed questions by governors and enabling periodic review at regional and national levels; and to attempt some initial, tentative links between resources and regime delivery. The system requires governors systematically and regularly to collect information about the delivery of key services, activities, and routines in a form that could be directly related to the components of the individual functions document, i.e. data are recorded daily, collated in a weekly report, and are available to the governor on the following Monday.

There are six component groups to the weekly data sheet. First, actual and planned weekly figures for inmate hours, inmate numbers, and staff operating hours are compiled across twelve categories of inmate occupation including time spent on various educational activities, workshops, catering, farm work, gardening, induction, and miscellaneous occupations. Second, the planned and actual inmate hours spent in physical education, evening education, and chaplaincy activities. Third, a simple checklist of eight successfully completed routines comprising canteen, exercise, bathing, association, kit change, mail distribution, library time, and receiving visits. Fourth, other indicators provide more detail about certain routines – the time spent in libraries, official and domestic visits, or completed petitions. Fifth, there is space for operational comments regarding issues such as breaches in security, the number and type of incidents, and about catering problems. Last, the daily average number of hours spent outside the cell on weekdays and weekends is sampled.

Clearly, the weekly monitoring system represents a radical improvement in the way the prison service records data about its activities. With the exception of one or two input measures, the system essentially consists of a set of activity measures that can be used to assess the performance of individual regimes against the targets agreed in the functions document. A quality dimension is implicit in many of the PIs because of the information that they provide about the nature of prison life, such as the number of hours inmates spend outside their cell and on activities. This information supplements the role of the Inspectorate in monitoring quality which is particularly useful for senior management, given that the inspectorate has the resources to visit establishments on average no more than once every eight years. One way of extending the capacity of the system to evaluate quality and effectiveness would be to adopt Dunbar's (1985) suggestion that the prison service should do more than count what the organisation provides in terms of the number of activities; it should also produce disaggregated data on what each individual actually receives. This would also represent a way of incorporating the impact of the service on the consumers (if the consumers are taken to be the inmates); as it is they have no input.

The weekly monitoring system is an important instrument of organisational control. As one regional director put it: 'We are the managers and we developed the regional monitoring system. We see a need for performance indicators as a means of control over what our governors are doing.' The system increases control over regime performance in two important ways: the functions document fixes baselines which are, effectively, negotiated performance targets; and the standardised data set allows the region to make time-series comparisons of individual regime performance and comparisons between different regimes. But the benefits are not felt exclusively at regional level; as we shall see, the monitoring system has enhanced the capacity of managers of individual establishments to obtain greater knowledge about and control over the performance of their own regimes. In short, performance review is improved by the availability of better information at all levels of the service: the individual regime reviews both weekly and monthly; the region reviews monthly and quarterly; and there are national reviews quarterly and annually. In principle, these reforms should have reinforced accountability at every level of the organisation.

The weekly monitoring system is purpose-built. Unlike most other public sector systems it is not a 'data-driven' system. It does use some existing data, for example educational and workshop activities have long been measured, but a large amount of new data is also generated. Moreover, these new data are collected for the specific purpose of constructing useful performance indicators. Many of these PIs are *negative* indicators because the assumption underlying the monitoring system is that the PIs should operate as alarm-bells that warn managers of potential problems. For example, it is accepted that there is a link between serious discontent among inmates and the failure of the prison authorities to carry out certain basic routines; hence the simple checklist recording whether eight core activities, such as the regular distribution of mail or the opportunity to have a bath, have been carried out satisfactorily. The logic is straightforward; the governor can monitor these negative PIs for a warning about whether the conditions exist for a 'roofs off' situation to arise.

The system also has the rare merit (in the public sector) of being both timely and flexible. It is timely because it provides reliable measures of key regime components on a weekly basis. This quick snapshot of performance enables the governor to spot problems rapidly and to implement a quick remedial response; the system represents the contemporaneity of a newspaper rather than the detailed record of a historical textbook. It is flexible because it consists of a few key indicators rather than a vast number of PIs on the lines of the police matrix of indicators. This parsimony is particularly important for an information system that is updated on a weekly basis and for a monitoring system that is designed to be used as a day-to-day tool of management: if the burden on the collator is too great then the reliability of the data might suffer; if the output is a mass of intimidating statistics then the busy governor is unlikely to use it. The most satisfactory explanation for the timely and flexible nature of the system would appear to be the almost unique pressure on the prison service to respond rapidly to a breakdown in performance: if things go wrong in the police service then it may take some time before the repercussions are felt; in a prison the flames may be ignited immediately.

Not surprisingly, by attempting to create a flexible system, the designers have run up against criticism and opposition. There is suspicion among governors about the reliability of the PIs, fuelled by the cynicism arising from a tradition of poor management systems and by the newness of the weekly monitoring system. These worries are partly justified by the slow progress made since a computerisation programme was introduced during 1988; a combination of technical and staffing problems has impeded the development of a reliable information system. Despite these reservations, the indicators are intended to be a tool of day-to-day management. For this purpose senior administrators argue that it is less important that the PIs should be totally accurate than that they point managers towards problems that require remedial action: 'the indicators may be still low on reliability but they are a *way in* to asking questions about performance'; in short, they are tin-openers.

Some prison governors remain sceptical. It is argued that basing the PIs on activities means that they are poor proxies of output; how can the non-performance of certain tasks be directly linked to outbursts of violence? They also reject the need to adopt such quantitative techniques. As one senior enthusiast for the system argued, 'the most effective managers are "hands-on" managers. When I visit a prison I have a feel for how it is being managed; if the people are tense, if there is flexibility.' Certainly several governors reacted against the weekly monitoring system when it was first introduced; some even tried to change the form to make it more appropriate to the needs of their own establishment. Although governors recognised that the weekly monitoring system gave them greater control over their own establishment, some feared that it would be used by regional management to reduce the autonomy that governors have traditionally enjoyed. Specifically, governors disliked the monitoring system being used to compare the performance of individual regimes on the grounds that they are all so different. In recognition of this problem clusters of regimes have been isolated as a means of making national level comparison more valid (see Table 3.5). There are difficulties with this approach but as one manager commented: 'someone has to ask why establishments perform differently'.

The real obstacle to acceptance may be that governors do not want to know the answers to such questions because of the implications for their own management of their workforce. Do they want to read that, for example, costs vary widely both between and within the four regions? Thus in 1985–6 the south-east region had an average weekly net operating cost per inmate that was 17 per cent above that of the

Table 3.5 Average weekly hours of inmate activity delivered per inmate and average numbers of inmates involved in regime activities: April–September 1989

Type of establishment	Hours	Per cent of population (1)
Closed prisons (male)	24.99	79
Open prisons (male)	34.36	91
Remand centres and local prisons (male)	13.27	47
Young Offenders Institutions (male)	26.08	83
Female (training)	29.23	89
Female (local/remand)	18.45	59
All establishments	21.00	n/a

(1) Figures exclude time spent by inmates on association, physical exercise, or attending court.
Source: HM Treasury (1990), Cmnd. 1009

northern region, but of the three dispersal prisons in the northern region, one had costs 55 per cent higher than the cheapest, and one category-three training prison had costs five times greater than the average (Lord 1987: 40).

The prison service lagged behind most other departments in developing systems for measuring and evaluating organisational performance, yet it eventually constructed a quite innovative set of activity-based PIs. In short, it has a system of performance evaluation that, in contrast to the courts and, particularly, the police, is purpose-built, parsimonious, and timely. With these attributes, and by using negative indicators as tin-openers, the governors' weekly monitoring system is potentially an extremely effective instrument of day-to-day management. Underlying this system are three important features.

First, unlike all the organisations – public and private – examined in this book, the motivation for developing this system came from regional managers rather than the centre (something that one might have expected from a more decentralised organisation like the police). This makes it more likely that PIs will be actively used as a managerial tool because they were designed for that specific purpose. Second, the source of the conceptual breakthrough was the decision to focus on *process* – the way in which inmates are treated – rather than to pursue the more elusive, indefinable output measures. Third, by concentrating on process, regional managers are able to generate useful information about what their staff are actually doing, so that the Governor's Weekly Monitoring System, along with the Fresh Start agreement, forms a central part of a strategy for increasing managerial control over the workforce.

This is not to say that the prison service has resolved all its problems successfully; far from it, the new costing systems, the move to local budgeting, and the 'Fresh Start' agreement have all encountered serious implementation constraints. Moreover, despite the establishment of the functions document and the introduction of the monitoring system, the links between resource allocation and service delivery remain tenuous. But although it is still rather early to assess the extent to which the monitoring system and the performance indicators have been integrated into management practice, nevertheless it is apparent that management at all levels is now better equipped to monitor performance.

4   The welfare system

Social Security and the National Health Service

This chapter examines two organisations which are conventionally seen as delivering much the same kind of goods, i.e. tax-financed welfare, but which in practice turn out to be different in almost every respect. They are the Social Security system and the National Health Service.

SOCIAL SECURITY

Of all our public sector case studies, the Department of Social Security (DSS) appears to face the least problems in assessing its perform-ance, for its primary objective – the prompt and accurate processing of benefit claims – lends itself to straightforward measurement and evaluation.

Social Security provides a vast and wide-ranging service: the regional organisation deals with some 23 million callers each year through a network of almost 500 local offices employing some 70,000 staff, with approximately 10,000 staff employed in the other DSS agencies which are the Resettlement Agency, the Information Technology Services Agency, and the Contributions Unit (NAO 1988). It is a public sector, non-trading, monopoly with a completely 'captive market', for the DSS faces competition (from local councils and citizens advice bureaux) only in its function of informing the public about their entitlements to benefits.

The DSS is subject to the normal processes of departmental parliamentary accountability which will alter little after the transfer of most of the DSS to agency status in 1991. In practice, despite this straightforward relationship, the degree and nature of public scrutiny differ slightly from its former departmental stablemate, the higher profile NHS. In particular, during the first two Thatcher Administrations the emphasis within the media reporting of welfare payments tended to focus on 'dole scroungers', whereas in recent years the introduction of the social fund and cash limits has generated greater sympathy for the plight of the poor. Less attention is given to the administration of Social Security than to the NHS; when public interest is drawn it tends to be in a negative way such as by the exposure of fraudulent claims.

Social Security is a 'caseload' department; although the organisation delivers a number of different benefits, the product is essentially uniform, i.e. the payment of cash benefits to legitimate claimants. This primary concern with money-shuffling provides an easily identifiable and quantifiable output that represents the currency of evaluation. The basic objective of the organisation is clear: benefits should be paid quickly and accurately to claimants; if this is done then administrative effectiveness is achieved (although broader programme objectives such as the alleviation of poverty may require quite different means of evaluation). There are exogenous factors that affect the performance of individual offices: in particular, a heavy workload, an often hostile public, and a competitive white collar labour market may result in a very high staff turnover in certain city offices which would normally be detrimental to performance, but this is not the same type of conceptual uncertainty that characterises the NHS or the police. Moreover, the skills required of staff are largely similar and interdependence between different parts of the organisation is generally low, although the payment of non-contributory benefits such as income support does draw on a number of staff in different sections. The organisation has a conventional centralised hierarchical structure that limits the amount of discretion available to unit managers: there are strict rules for allocating staff based on tasks that are standardised, routinised, and which adhere to strict legally based procedures. In contrast to all the other public sector organisations covered in this book, the DSS has no powerful professional or employee groups, although pockets of strong trade union organisation do exist.

Put simply, Social Security is low on heterogeneity, complexity, uncertainty, and autonomy, but high on authority. Consequently, despite the size of the organisation, we might anticipate that performance measurement in Social Security would be more straightforward than in the other non-trading public sector organisations studied in this book.

The design and use of Social Security performance indicators

It is therefore not surprising that among government departments Social Security has a comparatively long tradition of performance measurement: it introduced its first set of PIs as far back as the early 1970s in response to the Fulton Report. A number of government departments developed new systems of performance measurement following Fulton but enthusiasm soon waned and only Social Security and Inland Revenue continued the Management by Objectives initiative beyond 1972 (Garrett 1980). Why Social Security carried this experiment further than most departments is partly lost in the mists of administrative history, but it is clear that when Management by Objectives (MBO) was first considered many inside the service were concerned by falling standards that were attributed to inadequate management control systems and the increasing size of local offices (Walton 1975). Given that performance measurement is easier in caseload organisations that are involved in processing a multitude of definable transactions, and given that Social Security has always been characterised by a more managerial than administrative organisational style (Garrett 1980), it is understandable why Social Security was interested in managerial reform.

The outcome was a 'Participative Management' scheme based on the principles of MBO which in form, if not practice, remains largely unchanged today. Briefly, the main elements of this system were a management structure that provided direct accountability from local to head office, a management information system, performance indicators, target-setting, and an annual performance review process (see Walton 1975; Matthews 1979). However, performance measurement provoked considerable opposition from trade unions, so despite being fully integrated into the organisational structure, managers recalled that performance measurement 'went backstage until resurrected by the FMI'. Even when the FMI arrived, senior management appeared unhurried in its response, as illustrated by a rather self-satisfied contribution to an early FMI progress report written in August 1984 which boasted that 'the local office performance indicator system provides an example of a well established system' (HM Treasury 1986a). Reference was made to ongoing work on developing measures of quality of service and some more sophisticated PIs but little sense of urgency was detectable. As one official commented, 'when the FMI came in, top management thought we had been doing it for years'.

The isolation of inputs and outputs is quite straightforward in Social Security: staffing levels and costs are the main inputs, the number of benefits paid is the basic output. However, it has proven difficult to relate inputs to outputs. Instead, the long-established system of PIs focused on the production of two basic output measures. The first was clearance time, a workload indicator measuring the amount of work cleared (i.e. the number of cases) as a percentage of the total amount of work available over a defined period (previously four weeks, now one calendar month). The second PI assessed the accuracy of payments by calculating the proportion of incorrect payments found in a regular managerial check on a 2 per cent sample of contributory and non-contributory benefits. These PIs were applied to key benefits in contributory and non-contributory work – sickness, maternity, retirement, and income support (formerly Supplementary Benefit) – along with associated visits, assessments, and general work on National Insurance contributions (see Tables 4.1 and 4.2). In contrast to our other public sector organisations, these PIs provided a good measure of effectiveness; what was less clear (or more contestable) was the level representing acceptable performance.

These PIs were not comprehensive for although speed and accuracy of payment are a fundamental part of service delivery they do not tell the whole story. Thus, until recently, the PIs covered only about half of local

Table 4.1 Social Security performance indicators: clearance times (in days)

	1984–5	1985–6	1986–7	1987–8	1988–9
Retirement pension claims	47	31	27	25	22
Sickness/invalidity benefit claims	11	10	10	10	10
Maternity benefit claims	15	13	12	17	15
Attendance allowance claims	45	42	44	41	38
Mobility allowance claims	53	46	40	40	40
Family credit					17
Income support claims					5
Supplementary benefit claims (excluding caller claims)	6	8	7	6	
Supplementary benefit caller claims	2	2	2	2	
Income support visits (all grades)					11
Supplementary benefit home visits by executive officers	10	10	9	10	
IS/supplementary benefit assessments reviewed	2	2	2	2	2
Income support appeals					20
Supplementary benefit appeals	–	18	21	23	
Child benefit: straightforward claims	4	6	4	6	4
One parent benefit claims	9	18	11	11	10

Source: HM Treasury (1990), Cmnd. 1014

Table 4.2 Social Security performance indicators: error rates (percentage of payments incorrect)

	1984–5	*1985–6*	*1986–7*	*1987–8*	*1988–9*
Short term contributory benefits	3.2	3.9	3.9	4.1	4.0
Attendance allowance	4.2	3.1	3.5	0.8	0.7
Mobility allowance	1.6	1.1	1.5	1.1	2.6
Family credit					8.6
IS/supplementary benefit	9.6	10.5	10.4	11.6	9.1
Child benefit	0.9	0.8	0.7	1.1	1.1
One parent benefit	5.6	4.5	3.8	4.0	4.1

Source: HM Treasury (1990), Cmnd. 1014

office work, although this has since been expanded to some 75 per cent by monitoring overpayments and fraud work. Local managers admitted that the omission of broad areas of office work encouraged them to concentrate on measurable tasks at the expense of non-measured items and provided an incentive to 'fiddle' the figures. Staff complained that key items, such as telephone work, are ignored: the volume of telephone traffic is not recorded yet it can interfere significantly with the efficient completion of primary tasks (it could also be an interesting negative PI hinting at the breakdown of another part of the system – a missing file, an inaccurate payment, etc.). However, it would of course be very difficult to measure telephone traffic because of the technical problem of allocating the ownership of performance between different functions, particularly in the case of non-contributory benefits which usually require several support activities and necessitate a number of PIs just to monitor one job. Staff absenteeism and turnover were not included in the formal monitoring system but they could be useful negative indicators pointing to low morale and hence poor performance: 'annual wastage for one key clerical grade in 1986-87 was 21 per cent in the bottom thirty performing offices compared with 5 per cent in the top thirty' (NAO 1988: 24). Nonetheless, Social Security clearly benefited from having a system that provided a reasonably wide coverage with a minimum of PIs.

Yet in practice the PI system was poorly used. This was largely due to the hierarchical nature of the monitoring system which because of the aggregation of 'broad-based averages' meant that 'the basic structure was tailored more towards providing summary information at senior levels than to that of relevant and accurate information at local levels' (Birch 1989). The aggregated averages that appear in the annual White Paper were certainly used at a strategic level in negotiations with

Ministers (although it is interesting to note that the published PIs have rarely been taken up in a parliamentary question, despite the often poor record of performance that they report). However, lower down the hierarchy, although information about PIs was reported monthly by local offices to the region and regularly passed up the line, there was very little feedback of information to local managers: they had access only to data about the other offices in their group within which perhaps only one or two offices faced comparable problems. Consequently, local office managers often attributed little importance to the compilation of data, illustrated by the tendency to delegate this task to junior or inexperienced staff (NAO 1988: 21), raising questions about the validity of the data and indicating that PIs were of peripheral importance to the day-to-day tasks of a local manager.

Moreover, much information was discarded as it filtered up the hierarchy so that local office data were generally unavailable at headquarters: the management board received national figures and certain regional figures; the director of the regional organisation looked at regional figures; the regional controller examined the group figures; and the group manager compared local office data. There was some flexibility in the system: 'we have a monthly meeting of the director and the seven regional managers. If a regional controller says that his bad figures are caused by five bad offices then the director can obtain the necessary data.' Nevertheless senior managers admitted that because only highly aggregated data were available at the centre it was impossible to monitor performance accurately. This was confirmed by the NAO (1988) which discovered that a marked variation in performance between offices was disguised by this aggregation. To illustrate, in 1986–7 clearance times for retirement benefit ranged from 14 to 57 days for different offices, with inner city offices generally performing worst (see Table 4.3). More specifically, the NAO found that 21 per cent of supplementary benefit claims were taking longer than ten working days to process: a situation that directly exacerbated the financial hardship of claimants and indirectly impaired organisational performance by

Table 4.3 Clearance times (in days) 1986–7

	National average	Individual office average	
		Best	*Worst*
Retirement pension	26	14	57
Supplementary benefit	6	2.5	15

Source: NAO (1988), 11–12

increasing the workload on offices in the form of written complaints, telephone enquiries, and personal visits to offices. Similarly, the NAO found that the degree of accuracy in supplementary benefits payments varied between 4.1 per cent and 25.4 per cent although the national average was 9.5 per cent. The aggregation of data also precluded the construction of meaningful league tables of offices at national level; where crude league tables did exist they were at group or regional levels.

It is therefore hardly surprising that, although some target-setting was introduced into Social Security in the early 1970s it was ineffectual. The introduction of 'participative management' had envisaged a twice-yearly review of staff and target achievement which would be fed up the line to reveal standards and planned improvement. In practice, staff recall that these intentions suffered from a number of constraints, both organisational, notably powerful trade union opposition, and political: after the early days of the Heath Administration there was a marked decline in interest in performance measurement. Even the subsequent formalisation of target-setting throughout the organisation in 1982 had little impact. Robin Birch, an under-secretary in the DSS, has observed that these were rather arbitrary and uninformative targets: 'the performance indicators tended to be regarded as targets, and therefore reflected what the organization, not under particular pressure, had done previously' (Birch 1989). These targets were set on a bottom-up basis: local managers decided what they could achieve, subject to some renegotiation with group managers ('bottom-up' did not encompass non-managerial staff). The targets were subsequently broken down into individual targets for line managers and staff within each office. Higher up, regional managers simply informed the director of the regional offices what they could achieve, 'these were very much regional targets; there was no analysis at the top'. Indeed, senior management now confesses that 'there was no planned progression built into the process . . . we had a process essentially descriptive in character which we sometimes described as a target-setting process though it was nothing of the kind' (Birch 1989).

This system of performance evaluation was used, largely unaltered, until the late 1980s when a number of developments undermined the complacency within the organisation regarding the need to respond to the FMI. Throughout the decade there was mounting criticism about the quality of service to the public that was highlighted by two critical reports from the National Audit Office (1988) and the Public Accounts Committee (1988). This exposure had a profound impact within the service: 'the NAO report has shaken us all up. It caused a big stir. We now see the deficiencies that we did not see before. It was a useful tool for change, for overcoming resistance.' The DSS was galvanised into commissioning an extensive and hard-hitting internal review, *The Business of Service*, which was adopted as the framework for transforming Social Security into agency status (Moodie *et al.* 1988). A central assumption underlying this report was that Social Security needed to adopt a more consumerist ethos. This reorientation was captured by the rather grand assertion that because of its functions of paying benefits and pensions, and receiving National Insurance contributions, 'Few organisations can have a greater claim to be a consumer organisation. Social security is a service which at some point or another, in some form or another, touches the whole population in ways that are uniquely personal and intimate' (Moodie *et al.* 1988: 3). More succinctly, 'Social security is in the business of service. Its product is good quality service.'

The unfolding story of poor organisational performance revealed two serious weaknesses in the system of performance evaluation. First, the message from the various reports was that PIs were not integrated into management systems and were therefore not being used as a tool for pinpointing and rectifying poor performance; in particular, the target-setting system was ineffectual. Second, there was the familiar absence of PIs that measured the quality of service. Quite clearly, the system of performance monitoring that had survived, subject to minor changes, for some fifteen years needed revamping.

The Business of Service report was quite explicit that the means of improving the first problem was to give paramount importance to the design and implementation of targets throughout the organisation; the subsequent adoption of this strategy illustrated that targeting was, as one senior manager put it, 'the flavour of the moment'. Thus when the Permanent Secretary admitted weaknesses in the previous system to the Public Accounts Committee – 'There has been a tendency for us to perhaps accept too readily targets that were proposed by those who were going to deliver them and that a slightly tighter discipline is required' (1988: para. 4507) – he was safe in the knowledge that the first set of national performance targets had just been introduced for the forthcoming year 1988–9 (just ten days before the PAC met!) as evidence that corrective action had been taken.

The new Social Security targets covered eleven benefits and related aspects of those benefits which are classified in terms of importance as 'key benefits' and 'other major areas' (see Table 4.4). These targets raised important questions. Previously the bottom-up targets had been operational; i.e. they indicated the improvement in performance that management expected, based on a calculation from the figures of the previous year. The introduction of national targets implied something quite different. Did they represent a standard that every office was expected to achieve, or merely one that would be tolerated? The Permanent Secretary stated that the targets would set a standard 'at a level which we judge to be achievable with effort' (PAC 1988: para. 4557). More specifically, Robin Birch explained that:

> We decided to set ourselves a long-term target performance (which we describe as the 'desirable' target) and a short-term 'minimum tolerable' standard. We have set ourselves a period of three to four years in which to progress through the 'minimum tolerable' standard and up to that which we describe as 'desirable'.

Although all performance will be monitored, 'managerial efforts at least at the outset, will be concentrated on bringing those offices which are not even performing at the minimum tolerable level up to that standard as a start' (Birch 1989). In other words, as Table 4.4 shows, Social Security is adopting a cautious, exception-reporting approach aimed at eliminating the poorest performers.

The uniform national standards were not broken down into specific targets for individual offices which prevented any account being taken of the various environmental factors that influence the performance of individual offices. Thus although branch managers could now assess their performance against a national standard, it remained questionable how useful these targets were when it was impossible to make a

Table 4.4 Targets for the Social Security regional organisation

Targets in working days unless otherwise stated	Tolerable range	Targets 1989–90	Targets 1990–1	Targets 1991–2
SF crisis loans	0–1	1	1	0
IS claims	3–5	5	4	4
IS error rate	5–9%	9%	8%	7%
IS assessment review	2–3	3	3	2
SF community care grants	5–10	8	7	6
SF budgeting loans	5–10	8	7	7
SB/IVB claims	7–12	10	9	9
CB error rate	3–5%	3.7%	3.5%	3.5%
RP claims	18–27	24	23	22
RP load	12–15	13	13	13
Contributory files	25–40	36	34	32
Contributory pouches	16–28	25	24	23

Source: Secretary of State for Social Security, 17 May 1989 (DSS)
Notes: SF = Social Fund; IS = income support; SB = sickness benefit;
IB = invalidity benefit; CB = contributory benefits; RP = retirement pension.

like-with-like comparison with offices of equivalent size operating in similar circumstances. Consequently, the PIs were still being used as 'tin-openers' rather than 'dials'; a point illustrated by the Permanent Secretary when discussing a particular office that produced a seven days clearance rate for income support when the target was for five days clearance:

> We have to ask ourselves why that happened; this is the normal management process. It may be because the office is just incompetent. It may be because the office had a particular event in the area which caused the work to be set back. It may be because we knew at the start that the office would not achieve it because it is an inner London office but we wanted to set them something they could aim at.
>
> (PAC 1988: para. 4562)

The PIs cannot be used as dials without a more sophisticated information system that would allow like-with-like comparisons.

Work is under way to resolve this problem by developing 'aggregate PIs' that, in addition to the existing measures of throughput and accuracy, would cover productivity, pressure of work on offices, the time taken to clear an office of work, and an indicator that weights office workload according to the individual mix of activities. For example, the aggregate productivity PI provides the ratio of input to output in local offices, and another measures the 'balance' between clearance, accuracy, and productivity. These aggregate PIs would overcome the problem of differing environmental circumstances: the case-mix of an office – the weighting of contributory against the more complex non-contributory benefit work – would be taken into account, as would the impact of staffing shortages and high turnover in dangerous or undesirable inner city offices, and the extra work generated by seaside bed and breakfast claims. To allow valid comparisons to be made, clusters of offices will be constructed using variables such as inner city, rural, seaside, rather than simply office size. If this experimental package proves successful it would represent an important breakthrough, enabling national targets to be broken down into targets for individual offices: as one enthusiast explained, 'it will allow us to hold local offices responsible by saying that after all the variables have been "normalized" then you should achieve "x" ... and then we can go on to make the crucial link to resources'. However, although it is possible to set basic productivity targets, the shortage of financial unit cost PIs, due to the conceptual and technical difficulties of apportioning staff time to specific tasks, still prevents the construction of reliable efficiency measures for individual offices and functions.

Compared with many other public sector organisations the second problem – the lack of quality PIs – might appear rather strange, given the availability of two reasonably robust effectiveness measures – clearance times and error rates. Moreover, since 1984 there has also existed a constitutional system of performance evaluation represented by the office of the Chief Adjudication Officer who has a statutory obligation to monitor the standards of adjudication of claims and to report to the Secretary of State for Social Security. The government reform of the adjudication process was, in the words of Tony Newton, Minister for Social Security, intended 'to improve the independence, quality and consistency of the adjudication process' (Sainsbury 1989). The Adjudication Officer is responsible for dealing with many of the complaints about Social Security by safeguarding due process and ensuring that claims are dealt with correctly and accurately. The Chief Adjudication Officer inspects forty-two local offices annually, scrutinising decisions in a sample number of cases, examining the routine office monitoring checks and the appeals preparation work (Sainsbury 1989). Where the adjudication work is found to be inadequate a 'comment' will be made. This comment may be substantive – such as an incorrect application of the law – or procedural – a mistaken record of the decision. The comments total is then disaggregated according to the type of benefit and from these figures various PIs can be constructed. A basic PI is the 'comment ratios' – the percentage of claims for which at least one adjudication comment is raised – which can be used as a crude measure of adjudication performance. However, Sainsbury finds no evidence that standards of adjudication have improved since 1984 and he argues that the Chief Adjudication Officer commands little respect within the service – office monitoring teams are 'often perceived as "nit-picking"'. In particular, a major problem is the absence of explicit standards by which to judge the quality of adjudication. Nevertheless the Chief Adjudication Officer represents a potentially important mechanism for monitoring and controlling the quality of service.

However, the widespread criticisms of service quality has focused on issues of *process*: such as the length of time that claimants had to wait in benefit offices, the inhospitable condition of the surroundings, and the poor service offered by sullen, unhelpful staff. Neither the effectiveness PIs nor the Chief Adjudication Officer provided a clear picture of process: the DSS simply lacked the capability to assess these aspects of service delivery. The solution was to develop a 'Quality Assessment Package' (QAP) (see Table 4.5) which regularly measured waiting times and carried out a periodic postal questionnaire survey of customer opinion to monitor the length of waiting time endured by clients, delays

Table 4.5 Quality of service statistics 1988–9

	Income support/ Social Fund	Contributory benefits
(1) *Caller times*		
Pre-reception waiting times (average)	11.6 mins	7.9 mins
Total time spent in the office (average)	19.6 mins	14.5 mins
Satisfactory standard of interview achieved	92 %	93 %
(2) *Visits*		
Satisfactory standard of interview achieved	89 %	–
(3) *Outgoing mail*		
Satisfactory standard achieved	45 %	74 %

Source: HM Treasury (1990), Cmnd. 1014

in visiting, and the standard of interviewing and of correspondence in a sample of twenty-one local offices. The QAP was first included in the Public Expenditure White Paper in 1985, albeit in a highly aggregated form and providing no figures for earlier years or any statement about desired standards of service; in short, it provided little useful knowledge. Furthermore, the accuracy of the QAP was questioned widely within the service; a suspicion that was verified by an NAO-commissioned Gallup poll that found a significantly larger number of claimants to be seriously dissatisfied with local office service than was revealed by the QAP (subsequently the DSS decided to commission regular independent customer research). Hardly surprising then that progress in developing and implementing this package was slow, with only three regions making even limited use of it by 1988 (PAC 1988: para. 4442). It was the rising tide of public criticism that forced the DSS to put more effort into improving the standard and use of this package. Thus, following a commitment to the PAC that all offices would be operating the QAP by 1988–9 (PAC 1988: para. 4443), a more sophisticated version of the system was implemented in every office during that year (see Table 4.6). Subsequently, the coverage of this package was extended during 1989–90 and, significantly, the results of this package were fed into the target-setting process during 1990–1, targeting three key quality PIs for the first time: caller waiting times, quality of correspondence, and quality of interviews.

It is perhaps surprising that Social Security found itself the object of so much criticism about its methods for measuring performance, given that it is a caseload organisation that is low on heterogeneity, complexity, and uncertainty, and, moreover, has a history of using

Table 4.6 Quality Assessment Package 1989–90

Caller waiting times	
Quality of interviews	
Quality of correspondence	} by continuous assessment
Quality of telephone service	
Delays in issuing renewal order books	
Customer perception of the service provided	
Number of violent incidents in public areas of the office	
Facilities provided by the office for the public	

Source: DSS internal document (1989)

performance measurement that stretches back for almost two decades. Criticisms of its performance have highlighted deficiencies in its evaluation system; namely the lack of quality PIs and the absence of an explicit, credible set of performance standards. Yet, ironically, the system of performance measurement, replete with a set of output measures that captured some 75 per cent of performance in around twenty PIs, was probably at least as impressive as the other public sector organisations in our study. We might have expected such a parsimonious and timely system to be widely used by local managers, particularly the negative indicators that quickly signal the existence of problems. In practice, the poor quality of data, the high degree of aggregation, and the ineffectual target-setting process meant that the PIs were held in rather low regard throughout the organisation.

However, it would be unwise to assume that the mounting criticism of Social Security simply reflected problems with the existing system of performance measurement. Rather Social Security was confronting new strains on the system – the rapid rise in unemployment and the transition to a new system of welfare benefits brought extra work without matching increases in resources – and facing new objectives, such as the need to respond to consumerist criticisms. Together these increased the visibility of Social Security to the public. Perhaps Social Security also suffered from not having the excuse of the police and prison services in the face of teething troubles that 'at least we are having a go'. Yet the speed with which Social Security management has responded to criticisms (accelerated by the transition towards agency status) is evident in the rapid extension of the Quality Assessment Package into every office and the imposition of national targets. This suggests that there are few insurmountable organisational obstacles to the development of a better system of performance measurement.

THE NATIONAL HEALTH SERVICE

Of all the organisations in our study, the National Health Service is by far the largest, most complex, and most heterogeneous. It is also the country's largest employer, with a total staff of 1,000,000. In turn, the staff covers an extraordinary range of expertise and specialisations. They include doctors and nurses, accountants and managers, remedial gymnasts and medical physicists, laboratory staff and cooks, cleaners and receptionists, physiotherapists and pathologists. The list could go on: many of the groups, notably the medical profession, splinter into a variety of sub-specialisations. Moreover, the very concept of 'delivering medical or health care' (if that is seen as the mission of the NHS) is elusive and difficult to define with any precision. Pragmatically, it consists of a catalogue of activities longer even than Leporello's recital of Don Giovanni's conquests, delivered in a large variety of settings. Hospitals may be delivering long stay or acute care; the form of acute care may vary from day surgery to dramatic displays of technological virtuosity in transplanting organs. Even in a general practitioner surgery, a very simple organisation when compared with a hospital, a variety of different activities is carried out. The point is obvious enough and hardly needs labouring: the NHS is a confusing ant heap of frenetic, but frequently uncoordinated sets of unrelated activities, which somehow add up to the delivery of health care to the entire population. Not only is it the largest organisation in Britain; it is the only one whose services are used by almost every woman, man, and child every year: in all, there are about 250 million contacts annually between the NHS (including general practice) and consumers.

Moreover, the NHS is an organisation where there is no 'bottom line'. This is obviously, and uninterestingly, true in the sense that as a tax-financed public service, the NHS makes no profits and declares no dividends. More importantly, for the purposes of our study, there is no way of summing up the myriad activities of the NHS or of translating these into a currency of evaluation which will allow the overall performance of the organisation as a whole to be measured from year to year. Not only are the activities of the NHS multiple. So are the NHS's objectives as set out, for example, by the 1979 Royal Commission (Merrison 1979: para. 2.6). These include ensuring equality of access and providing services of a high standard: objectives which may be in conflict with each other, given resource scarcity. What comes first: widening access, or improving standards for those who have already gained access? But, perhaps more fundamental still, the performance of the NHS cannot be measured in the terms which would appear to be most crucial: the impact on the health of the population. There has long been controversy about the extent to which medical intervention affects life expectancy and the available evidence suggests that nutrition, housing, and income have historically been more significant (McKeown 1979). And while there are plenty of reliable statistics about mortality, which tell us little or nothing about the performance of the NHS, there is a conspicuous famine of the morbidity data needed to tell us about the impact of the NHS on the quality of people's lives: as the Royal Commission argued (Merrison 1979: para. 3.16): 'the benefits of chiropody and hip replacements will not show up in the statistics but may make the difference between immobility and self-sufficiency for many old people'. In an important sense, therefore, the NHS's activities *are* its performance.

If the NHS appears to be unique in its size, complexity, and heterogeneity – as well as the uncertainty about the link between activities and impact (if any) – it is also an administrative oddity. From its birth in 1948, there has been tension between the doctrine of accountability to the centre and the fact of delegated responsibility to the periphery (Klein 1989b). As the man or woman responsible for the NHS, the Secretary of State for Health is clearly accountable to Parliament for everything that happens in the NHS since the service is financed out of public money. This is the famous bed-pan doctrine, as enunciated by Aneurin Bevan: 'if a bed-pan drops in any hospital corridor, the noise should reverberate through the corridors of Whitehall'. Yet, at the same time, given the scale and scope of the NHS, it has always seemed inconceivable that the whole operation should be run from the centre, just as it has been seen desirable that services at the periphery should be responsive to local needs and demands. Hence the baroque administrative structure of the NHS: service delivery in England is the responsibility of some 190 district health authorities, responsible to fourteen regional health authorities who, in turn, are responsible to the Secretary of State for Health. Quite separately, there are ninety Family Practitioner Committees, which administer the primary health care services and are responsible to the Department of Health. This structure is under modification following the publication of the Government's Review of the NHS (Secretary of State for Health 1989). But it provides the background for the evolution of the NHS performance review system, of which performance indicators were part, during the course of the 1980s; an evolution which, in many ways, can be interpreted as yet one more attempt to resolve the tension between agency and autonomy in the NHS.

Bevan, in 1948, was quite clear about the status of the various boards and committees that were responsible for running the NHS. These, he stressed, were simply the 'agents' of central government and, as such, responsible for carrying out its policies. And, indeed, if one could think about the NHS as an organisation which delivers its services through some 300 'branches', there would be nothing remarkable about it. The number of health authorities involved is, in fact, rather less than the number of branches in some of the other organisations covered by this study. What has hitherto distinguished the NHS 'branches', however, is the extent to which they have managed to claim *de facto* autonomy. In part, this stems from the difficulty of defining the objectives of the NHS and measuring its performance: a point already touched on which will be further developed in the specific context of the development of PIs. This difficulty compounds the problems of control common to all organisations. In part, however, it reflects two factors specific to the NHS. The first is the composition of the various NHS authorities and committees. Until the implementation of the 1990 National Health Service and Community Care Act, their membership always included representatives of local communities and of the professional providers. In turn, this quasi-representative role gave them a sort of autonomous legitimacy: accountability to the centre and responsiveness to the local community do not necessarily point in the same direction. The second is that the ability of these authorities and committees to be accountable for the services for which they are responsible is circumscribed by the autonomy of the NHS providers (Day and Klein 1987). Most conspicuously, the medical profession makes large claims to immunity from scrutiny in the name of clinical autonomy. The transmission-belt model of decision-making and accountability in the NHS has therefore never worked, and much of its political and administrative history in the 1970s and 1980s can be interpreted as a succession of attempts to resolve the tension between agency and autonomy, between managers and providers, between centre and periphery, and to bring the regional and district barons under control.

The design and use of performance indicators in the NHS

Central to all these complicated tensions is the role of information. Accountability presumes both the availability of information about what is happening, and agreement about how such information should be interpreted (Day and Klein 1987). Many of the concerns of the 1980s, and particularly those which helped to shape the developments of the PI system, reflect long-running themes. As early as 1956, the Committee of Enquiry into the Cost of the National Health Service (Guillebaud 1956: paras 350–1) called for a new accounting system in order to make the hospital service accountable and drew attention to the importance of 'establishing at the hospital and departmental levels a system of effective budgetary control which will enable hospital managements in suitable cases to set their standards of efficiency each year and to judge at the end of the year whether those standards have been achieved'. A decade later an ex-Minister of Health lamented:

> The attempts to find satisfactory measurements of yardsticks of performance have been persistently baffled. Enormous effect has been lavished during the twenty years of the National Health Service on the collection of statistics of hospital activity, and on the search among them for the means of making valid comparisons, within the service itself and between the service and the other systems. It is a search I myself engaged in with the freshness and hopefulness of inexperience only to be driven into recognising reluctantly that the search itself was inherently futile. The most carefully constructed parallels between one hospital or hospital group and another dissolved on closer examination into a baffling complex of dissimilarities. Every attempt to apply a common standard had the effect of disclosing a deeper level of individual differences and incommensurables.
>
> (Powell 1966: 52–3)

However, while the case for improved performance measurements had been eloquently made in the 1960s and 1970s, little had been done to produce them. So in explaining the rise of PIs in the 1980s, we have to examine what was different about the 1980s: a combination, as we shall see, of new technology and a new political and economic environment. This search for 'satisfactory measurements of yardsticks of performance' continued in the 1970s. For example, a Working Party – chaired by an economist who was later to be policy adviser to a Labour Secretary of State – argued for investment in a new information system. Specifically, it underlined the need for 'a measure of output – of the extent to which particular objectives have been attained'. It also drew attention to a problem which has already been touched on:

> Not the least of the difficulties to be overcome in improving standards of management and evaluating performance is that it has for so long been tacitly accepted within the NHS that the activities of the medical profession lie outside management control.
>
> (Abel-Smith 1973: 16)

The 1980s were marked by a sharp reversal in government policy towards the NHS (Klein 1985) which, to a large extent, provides the explanation for the rise of PIs. The start of the 1980s was marked, in line with the 1979 General Election manifesto, by enthusiasm for decentralisation. Patrick (subsequently Lord) Jenkin, the then Secretary of State, became the prophet of power to the periphery. It appeared that the NHS was on the point of becoming a loose federation of health authorities. His manifesto, *Care in Action* (Department of Health and Social Security 1981), proclaimed: 'Local initiatives, local discussions and local responsibility are what we want to encourage'. Within the year there had been a remarkable about-turn. A new Secretary of State, Norman Fowler, was in the process of introducing a new period of centralisation. And it was as part of this process of strengthening the DHSS's grip on the NHS – of stressing accountability to the centre, rather than delegation to the periphery – that a new system of performance review, complete with indicators, was introduced. In January 1982, Fowler told the House of Commons that in future Ministers would lead reviews of 'long term plans, objectives and effectiveness of each region' with regional chairmen and officers who, in turn, would 'hold their constituent district health authorities to account'. As part of this new system, the DHSS was planning to use 'indicators of performance in the delivery of health services' to 'enable comparison to be made between districts and so help Ministers and the regional chairmen at their annual review meeting to assess the performance of their constituent district health authorities in using manpower and other resources efficiently'.

The story, as subsequently told by the then Permanent Secretary of the DHSS (Stowe 1989), was short and simple. It started with a report from the House of Commons Committee of Public Accounts (1981) which was highly critical of the Department's failure to ensure adequate financial control and accountability. It identified, specifically, the need to 'monitor key indicators of performance by the regions'. From this flowed, in Sir Kenneth Stowe's version, the invention of the performance review system and the related development of PIs. In fact, the development of performance indicators as such seems to have had a rather more complex, and longer, lineage. The pressure on the Department had been building up for some time (Klein 1982). A year before the Public Accounts Committee report, the Social Services Committee (1980) had stung the Department by its criticism of the failure to collect adequate information about the link between expenditure levels and service provision. A Working Party, chaired by Edith Körner, to examine the entire data system of the NHS had been set up at the start of the decade. And in his evidence to the 1981 Public Accounts Committee, Sir Patrick Nairne – Stowe's predecessor as

Permanent Secretary – talked about using 'what the jargon would describe as performance indicators' to monitor the efficiency in the NHS.

So far the rise of the health care PIs has been discussed exclusively in the context of the NHS itself. But, of course, their development can only be understood in a wider context: specifically, the emergence of a new managerial culture in Whitehall, symbolised by the Financial Management Initiative. Departments had to demonstrate that they were using the latest management tools in order to carry conviction with the Treasury. Equally significant, perhaps, the NHS PIs were invented as an instrument of central control: as an answer to the criticism that the DHSS did not exercise enough control over what was happening at the periphery. Whereas Sir Patrick Nairne had stressed the role of information as a means for making health authorities more accountable to local communities, his successor emphasised its role in making those authorities more accountable to the centre. However, the contrast between the emphases of these two Permanent Secretaries provides a theme which has continued to run through the whole history of the PI experiment so far. Depending on the audience being addressed, the Department of Health (as the DHSS became in 1989) has tended to put a somewhat different gloss on the role of PIs. To its parliamentary critics, PIs have been presented as an instrument of departmental control and as a way of reinforcing accountability to the centre. To NHS managers and members, PIs have tended to be presented more as a tool of self-appraisal, as a way of seeing the performance of their own district within a national framework: a mirror for their own use, rather than as a threatening instrument of central interference.

The first package of performance indicators was published by the DHSS in September 1983 (Pollitt 1985). It was not the product of any considered strategy for developing a management information system for the NHS. It represented, rather, a mass baptism of existing statistics in what was, in effect, a rather hurried administrative expedient. Statistics that had been around in the NHS for decades suddenly emerged re-born and re-christened as performance indicators; indeed John Yates of the Health Services Management Unit at the University of Birmingham had long since pioneered the use of data as policy indicators. The set of PIs, as published, contained virtually no new information. The package was also, in the light of future developments, remarkably parsimonious in the amount of information provided. It used only about seventy indicators – a number which had risen, by 1989, to 2,500 – provided at the level of both individual districts and individual hospitals: PIs for Family Practitioner Committees were to be produced at a later stage, but are not referred to further in this analysis.

The composition of the package suggested three main policy concerns. First, there was the concern about the efficient use of NHS resources, as reflected in the PIs dealing with lengths of stay, throughput, and turnover intervals in hospitals: efficiency being defined in the narrow sense of intensive, rapid use. Second, there was concern about value for money, as reflected in the PIs breaking down the costs of treatment into their component parts – manpower, catering, etc. Third, there was concern about access to the NHS, as reflected in the PIs providing data about admission rates and waiting lists. Like the statistics themselves, these concerns were part of the NHS's history: the invention of PIs symbolised thus a new managerial style rather than representing any intellectual or political break-through.

Soon after the launch of the first 'crude' package, the DHSS set up a Joint Group to prepare a more sophisticated second version. The Group not only included technicians, academics (including one of the authors of this book), and civil servants but also a range of people drawn from the NHS, among them clinicians and a regional chairman. Its composition was thus intended to stress that the production of PIs should be seen as a common enterprise between the DHSS and the NHS, and that the new set should be perceived as acceptable and useful to those at the periphery instead of being viewed (and resented) as an intrusive and threatening instrument of central managerial control. The same approach was taken to the membership of sub-groups each charged with developing indicators for specific aspects of the NHS: e.g. manpower and estate management, acute services, and provision for the elderly. Everyone laboured mightily. And the result, unsurprisingly, was a multiplication of PIs: a breeding process that has continued ever since. The final package that emerged from the 1985 exercise contained some 450 PIs (Department of Health and Social Security 1986). However, it was distinguished from its predecessor in a number of important respects, numbers apart. First, the 1985 package moved from the Gutenberg era into the IT era: it was distributed on computer discs. Second, to make information more accessible, the PIs were presented hierarchically: the computer package put a number of key indicators on the screen which might, or might not, explain the first set of figures. Third, the 1985 model not only provided more detail but also extended the data about access to, and the availability of, services. For example, in the case of services for the elderly, the PIs provided some information about levels of provision in the community. Such was the commitment of the DHSS to the notion of PIs by this time that the package was launched even though a test run in one region had produced the advice that the whole exercise should be put on ice for a year.

Given this commitment, it is not surprising that PIs have since become institutionalised and routinised in the NHS. One innovation requires noting, however. When producing the 1988 package, the Department took a new initiative. It sent out a circular requiring all district health authorities to review their own PIs: an attempt to create a new local constituency for PIs by involving members. As part of this initiative a glossy, coloured booklet was produced (DHSS, 1988) which showed variations in district performances: so, for example, one map identified those districts where the proportion of its residents receiving acute in-patient treatment was between 25 per cent and 50 per cent above or 10 per cent to 25 per cent below the national average, while other maps showed variations in cost per case and lengths of stay. Further, it also showed trends over time: the changes in the distribution of PI between 1983 and 1986 – so making it possible to see whether variations between authorities were narrowing. Table 4.7 shows a selection of the indicators used. The booklet was quite clearly designed as an exercise in popularisation aimed at a new audience, with each map accompanied by a short blurb explaining how the information should be interpreted: thus, in a sense, it represented a reversion to Nairne's 1981 concept of using PIs as an instrument of accountability to the local community.

We conclude this short history of PIs in the NHS by looking briefly at the likely future of the system, as outlined in the report of the Health Service Indicators Group (1988). This successor to the 1983 Group had as its primary remit to bring together the existing PIs and the NHS's new Körner data sets into a new system. However, as before, much of the work consisted in mobilising support for the PI system by consulting widely about possible changes and drawing in a large cast of experts. For example, the bodies consulted about possible new indicators ranged from the Royal College of Surgeons to the General Municipal Boilermakers and Allied Trades Union – almost 100 organisations in total. Its specific recommendations included some interesting features. First, it proposed indicators linked to policy goals set by the Government, such as the number of hip replacements and coronary by-pass grafts carried out. Second, it introduced the notion of outcome indicators, i.e. standardised mortality ratios for residents of each district for a range of conditions, as well as hospital mortality rates. However, like the 1985 report, the 1988 one concluded that 'more work needs to be done' in developing measures of outcome and quality and thus remedying what, from the start, had been seen as one of the major weaknesses of the PI package (see below). More generally, the 1988 report identified one of the major dilemmas in the design and production of PIs in the NHS. If PIs are to be used as an instrument of

Table 4.7 Selected National Health Service performance indicators

Proportion of district's residents treated as acute in-patients

Number of days it would take to clear the district's waiting list for general surgery at current activity levels

District's costs per case compared to the national average for the specialty mix of cases treated

Average length of stay in different specialties compared with the national average, given mix of patients treated

Average number of patients treated per general surgery bed per year

Proportion of district's over-75 residents who were discharged from hospital or died there and who had spent more than six months as an in-patient

Proportion of the district's over-65 residents who had at least one contact with a district nurse during the year

Number of registered nurses in special care baby units as a ratio of the number of low weight babies born

Proportion of nurses providing care for mentally ill people who work in community based services

Proportion of total annual expenditure on staff which is attributable to each of the main staff groups (medical, nursing, professional and technical, administrative, ancillary)

Proportion of emergency ambulance calls which meet response time standards

Source: Taken from Department of Health and Social Security (1988) *Comparing Health Authorities*, London: DHSS

top-down monitoring or control, then it is important to ensure birth-control: a parsimonious set is required if Ministers, central managers, or even members are not to be drowned in data. If, however, PIs are to be seen as part of the managerial culture of the NHS as a whole, it is essential that the information should be seen as relevant by those using it locally: this suggests the development of yet *more* PI sets, as the report recommended, at the level of individual units and departments. No wonder then, perhaps, that the NHS performance indicator package looks set to expand, in line with the growing capacity of information technology to handle ever vaster sets of data and to distribute such capacity ever more widely in the NHS. Given the choice beween a limited, table d'hôte menu and an à la carte system of PIs, the NHS opted for the latter.

In analysing the impact of PIs on the NHS, there is one fundamental difficulty. This stems from the fact that the PIs are, as already noted, simply a way of packaging old statistics in a new form. It is the label on the package, not its contents, which is new. The label announces, as it were, that political and managerial importance is now attached to comparing the performance of different health authorities and the units within them. In itself, this is significant. It represents the assertion of a new managerial philosophy in Whitehall. What we do not know, and perhaps cannot know, is what difference this symbolic assertion has made to the use of comparative data in decision-making, whether in the Department of Health or at the local management level in the NHS. There is no systematic study of the situation before 1983 to provide benchmarks; nor would such a study be all that helpful, given that so much else has happened since (like the diffusion of IT and continuing pressure on resources) calculated to make even traditionally innumerate DHSS civil servants and NHS managers interested in figures. All that we can say with any confidence is that while comparative data – notably about costs, lengths of stay, and manpower inputs – have been widely used for twenty years or more in the NHS, it is a new experience to enter the office of a civil servant in the Department of Health and find a desk top computer on his or her desk able to call up such statistics on the screen: technology has revolutionised accessibility while the new managerial culture puts a premium on using the new facility. In short, the desk top computer symbolises a revolution in the management of the NHS (Day and Klein 1989), of which the production of PIs is only a symptom.

Certainly, as those responsible at the Department of Health see it, PIs are only part of the drive to improve management in the NHS. They are meant to make managers at all levels 'more information conscious'. Although they are drawn upon in the planning and review process, 'as a diagnostic tool' and as a 'handy, accessible source of data', they do not determine the agenda or the issues being addressed. They make it easier to test the realism of regional plans; they allow questions to be asked about large divergences between districts in a region. In this sense, PIs are becoming domesticated in the new management culture. However, they are less integrated into the annual review process than might have been expected from the circumstances of their birth. Nor is this surprising, perhaps. PIs, as frequently noted already, are shaped by available data. They are moreover historical data, hitherto two years out of date by the time they are published. The annual performance reviews are shaped by current, urgent political concern. Thus the notion of good performance inherent in the regional reviews is not necessarily related to what PIs can do or show. The regional reviews tend to be target-setting processes: so for example, regions may be asked to carry out a specified number of cardiac operations or to increase their facilities for renal patients (Day and Klein 1985). In short, the reviews are largely concerned with outputs. In this, they mirror the notion of good performance set out in the Public Expenditure White Paper (HM Treasury 1990: Cmnd. 1013). There, too, performance is defined in terms of achieving a set of output targets, such as the achievement of 14,000 bypass grafts, 70,000 cataract operations, and 50,000 hip replacements by 1990. Nor is this emphasis surprising: the government response to criticism about inadequate inputs to the NHS has been, consistently, to stress increasing outputs. It is thus politically imperative to bring about their achievement. Given this, it is not surprising that PIs, seen as a formal system rather than as a shorthand for making inform-ation more accessible, play a subsidiary role. They do not define 'good performance', but they do allow central decision-makers (and others) to explore the constraints on and the opportunities for achieving the government's policy targets.

Much the same picture emerges from interviews carried out at regional and district level. The PI package tends to be seen as a reference library, and a rather badly organised one at that, rather than as a routine management tool. In the words of one regional officer: 'If I were a manager on the ground, I would quickly find out problems because people would be beating on my door. Once a manager starts to rely on PIs on a day-to-day basis, they are in dead trouble. It means that they have no feel for the service.' It is not, therefore, PIs which identify or define problems; rather it is the existence of problems which usually prompt reference to PIs. For district and local managers, they may be used to bolster a case for more efficient use of existing resources. In short, the PI package seems to be used less for routine scanning or monitoring of performance (since this, as we have seen, is such an elusive concept anyway in the NHS and since data are not sufficiently timely to allow it to be used on such a day-to-day basis anyway) than as ammunition in the battle between the different levels of the managerial hierarchy. Furthermore, regions and districts – like the central department – are moving towards setting targets: so, for instance, regions will negotiate an agreed, achievable target with districts, where the same process will be carried out with unit managers, who in turn will set targets for reducing waiting lists or carrying out specific operations. Again, this implies using indicators linked to managerial targets, and devising local sets of PIs which are driven by local policy concerns rather than by the availability of a national data set. So the irony seems to be that the more successful the Department of Health becomes in carrying out its managerial revolution in the NHS, and making everyone more information conscious, the less need will there be for a national package of PIs since everyone will be able to design their own, tailored to their specific preoccupations and circumstances – all the more so since the new Körner data system will allow them to do so much more speedily and flexibly than any national package.

For given the political dynamics of the NHS, there are built-in incentives for any national PIs to be questioned at the local level, particularly if the data are used to challenge existing practices. The more the centre uses PIs as a means of scrutinising the local delivery of services, the more reason have the providers at the periphery to discredit the validity and reliability of potentially threatening information. And one of the distinguishing characteristics of the NHS is precisely that the key service providers, i.e. the medical profession, are certainly more highly trained and probably far more statistically numerate than those in the other organisations in our study. So, for example, when the regional health authority criticised the Department of Trauma and Orthopaedics at Kings's College Hospital, London, for low productivity, the response by the medical staff was to carry out an audit of their own activities (Skinner *et al.* 1988). They found that 'an exact classification and grading of operations' had led to an under-estimate of 34.5 per cent in the number of major operations per consultant. And they concluded that 'existing methods are too flawed to allow an accurate or meaningful assessment of performance'. In the 1990s, as in 1966, the NHS service deliverers not only have an incentive to demonstrate 'a deeper level of individual differences and incommensurables', to use Powell's words, but also considerable sophistication in so doing. In short, the persuasiveness and therefore usefulness of PIs may crucially depend on the local sense of ownership, based on an acceptance that they measure accurately – and in an agreed currency – the various dimensions of performance: they have to carry conviction with those whose work they are purporting to describe. And the more that PIs endeavour to measure what is actually happening at the point where NHS providers meet the patients – to convey a sense of what the service is actually like – the more important does this become.

The one national study of how the PI package has been used by health authorities (Jenkins *et al.* 1987) tends to confirm these conclusions, with one exception. It showed a 'fairly widespread use of PIs across a broad range of managerial activities': so, for example, 154 district general managers reported that PIs had been used in the regional review of their districts, as against only thirty-seven who said that they had not. In other words, PI-type information is indeed becoming an indispensable element of the managerial vocabulary in the NHS: 'part of the normal debating and politicking process within districts'. This study also confirms the view that the importance of the PI package, as distinct from information in a more general sense, was limited. It concluded that:

1 PIs were only part of the information used in a particular debate;
2 Use of PIs was reactive – information was usually sought once an issue had emerged rather than the consideration of PIs stimulating issues for the managerial agenda;
3 The PI information did not surprise managers but tended to confirm currently held views.

(Jenkins *et al.* 1987: 142)

The survey evidence did, however, suggest that there might be a continuing constituency for a national package of PIs, and this for two reasons. First, there was 'a general acceptance that performance can and should be assessed by comparison'. Second, many districts perceived 'few alternatives to PIs as a way of evaluating performance'. We therefore return to the conceptual problems of assessing performance in the NHS, and embodying that elusive notion in a set of PIs.

Inherent in the NHS system of PIs is a relative concept of performance, as already noted. There is no way of bringing together, in one dimension or in a single currency of evaluation, the many and various activities of the service. There is, above all, no way of measuring the combined impact of these activities on the health of the nation, as we have also seen. Given this lack of any absolute measures, it is inevitable that any set of NHS performance indicators has to fall back on second best, comparative indicators of performance. From this, however, flow a number of problems.

The first is that of defining the units of management or production where valid comparisons can be drawn. Thus the PI package provides data about districts and hospitals within them. But which of those districts, and which of those hospitals, are actually comparable? If District A treats fewer patients than District B then this might be because it is using its resources less intensively or because it has fewer resources or because it has a different kind of population with different needs for health care. If Hospital C has higher costs per patient than Hospital D, this might be because it is treating different kinds of patients, because its buildings are scattered around several sites, or because it is being incompetently managed. In short, the figures do not speak for themselves. As the Department of Health warned in its 1988 booklet:

The indicators are intended to raise questions and to highlight issues for further discussions and investigations in the light of local knowledge. They are not precise measures; nor do they cover all aspects of what health authority is responsible for ... No single indicator, or even group of indicators, can tell the whole story about a district's activities. They must always be considered in the light of more detailed local knowledge and information about the characteristics of individual districts.

(DHSS 1988: 7)

They are, in our vocabulary, tin-openers rather than dials. Only when they are linked to the achievement of specific, policy determined targets do they become dials off which it is possible to read 'good' or 'bad' performance – for implicit in such targets is a concept of absolute, rather than relative, levels of performance.

The claim to uniqueness of every NHS District and every NHS hospital (and every NHS consultant) can, of course, be challenged. Indeed the whole process of using PIs can be seen as a way of subjecting this claim to critical scrutiny and putting it on the rack of managerial examination. To a degree, changes in the technology of producing PIs also have a role to play in this: statistical skills can be used to narrow the scope for argument. So, for example, the PIs produced by the DHSS have from the first sought to standardise the statistics of cost, throughput, and length of stay for the case-mix: they compare, for each hospital, the actual composition of the case-mix. However, the various generations of PI sets so far produced have not addressed the question of the comparability of different districts. They have not followed the model of the Audit Commission, for example, which has produced 'clusters' or 'families' of local authorities which share the same socio-economic characteristics. In part, this may reflect the difficulty of deciding just what factors are important in distinguishing between health authorities: the inherited pattern of health facilities may be as important as socio-economic characteristics. It has therefore been left to individual districts to choose their own families: to decide in which comparative mirror they should examine their own performance. The logic of this is, of course, persuasive if PIs are seen as an instrument of managerial self-examination; it is rather less persuasive if they are seen as a way of making the periphery accountable either to the centre or to the community.

A further problem posed by a PI package based on comparisons is that it will, inevitably, draw attention to the outliers. That is, it prompts questions about those districts or hospitals which are conspicuously above or below the national average. This may be useful, in itself. But it does not tell us anything about the performance of those who are hidden in the pack, nor does it say anything about whether or not the national average represents a good or bad performance. Indeed even districts which perform above the national average on some criteria – for instance, the throughput of cases through beds or operating theatres – may not necessarily be setting an appropriate model for the rest: it could just be that their productivity is imposing too great a strain on their staff, and that as a result the quality of treatment is suffering.

To raise the question of quality is to point also to one of the main criticisms made of the PI package (for example, Pollitt 1985). This is that the emphasis of the PI package has consistently been on productivity and access, to the neglect of measures of quality outcome and consumer satisfaction. Both the 1985 and the 1988 Working Groups on indicators recognised this and, as we have seen, urged the development of appropriate measures to capture these extra dimensions. It is tempting to see this limitation on the scope of the PI package as deriving from the circumstances of its birth: the pressure within government generally to cut public spending, to squeeze more out of any given bundle of resources, and to achieve more value for money. Hence, of course, the suspicion at the time of the introduction of the first PI package that this was merely one more device to put pressure on NHS providers and to push up the statistics of activity, regardless of the effects on quality, outcome, or consumer satisfaction. However, even conceding that a concern about value for money provided much of the driving force behind the various managerial initiatives in the NHS, this would be a misinterpretation of what happened. The precise nature of the PI package was determined not by the preoccupations of the 1980s but by those of the 1950s, 1960s, and 1970s, i.e. the decades during which the NHS's system of collecting statistics had evolved. If the PI package concentrated excessively on costing and activity statistics, it was because these were the only statistics that were available. In short, much of the indictment of the PI system is an indictment of the NHS's whole history: its neglect of crucial dimensions of performance. The paradox is, rather, that a managerial preoccupation with getting more value for money and increasing productivity led to an interest in developing measures of quality, outcome, and consumer satisfaction that had been conspicuously lacking in previous decades. The fact that the search still continues, and has yet to produce a set of measures which can be used routinely to assess performance on these dimensions, in turn suggests that such indicators may be as difficult to design as they are desirable.

Organisational complexity and heterogeneity, a multiplicity of policy goals, and lack of agreement about how to measure performance have, in the NHS, led to a set of indicators conspicuous mainly for their propensity to proliferate. Add this to the fact that hitherto NHS performance indicators have been largely of historical interest by the time that they were published, and it is not surprising that they do not appear to have contributed much to major strategic or managerial decisions. They are a clear case of a PI package shaped by the availability of data rather than being designed to meet specific managerial requirements. Furthermore, it has never been quite clear whether they were intended to be an instrument of central control or managerial self-examination. The initial impetus for designing the package came from pressure to strengthen accountability to the centre; the continued interest in developing the package seems to derive more from a commitment to strengthen management throughout the NHS, and to persuade managers at all levels to look at their own performance. It is therefore difficult to disentangle the effects of introducing PIs from the wider changes in the managerial environment: in any case, their role and use will clearly change in the 1990s as the 1989 Review of the NHS (Day and Klein 1989) is implemented.

5 The private sector
Banks, building societies, and retail stores

We turn now to the private sector in order to examine how leading corporations and financial institutions make use of performance indicators. The chapter is divided into three main sections. The first compares the use of performance indicators in a major retail supermarket (Supermarket) and in a large high street retailer (HSR). The second draws on the experience of three financial institutions: one of the 'big four' clearing banks (Bank) and two leading building societies (Society X and Society Z). Lastly, there is a brief discussion of a TV rental, service, and sales company (Jupiter) which illustrates an interesting attempt to overcome the problems of measuring the performance of non profit-making branches within an organisation.

MANAGING A GOOD SHOP: SUPERMARKET AND HIGH STREET RETAILER

Supermarket and High Street Retailer (HSR) are, in many respects, very similar commercial organisations. Both are long-established national retail chains with several hundred outlets selling a wide variety of goods. Neither organisation faces great uncertainty because the single, dominant objective is to make profits, which is made easier by the clear relationship between processes, outputs, and outcomes: a well-run shop offering good quality, competitively priced goods backed up by sophisticated marketing should be profitable. In terms of both the number of stores and the range of goods, Supermarket and HSR are fairly heterogeneous and complex organisations – and have been getting more so, in both respects, over the last decade or so. Although both organisations operate in highly competitive environments, HSR in particular has been under considerable pressure to increase profits, lest there be a hostile take-over bid. The main differences between the two organisations are, however, that HSR manufactures many of the goods on its shelves and requires a greater range of expertise and marketing skills at the point of sale.

The most important similarity between the two organisations is that the overall level of profits, apart from establishing (in the long term) a reputation for being well-run shops, depends very largely on central decision-making, rather than on the managers of individual branches. The success of both businesses relies heavily on the efficient combination of several interdependent operations; the range and quality of goods on display is the result of orchestrating the relationship between the manufacturing (in the case of HSR), buying, distribution, and retail divisions. Supermarket has the pressure of dealing with food which is a perishable product possessing a relatively short shelf-life, but HSR has the additional complication of ensuring the efficiency of the manufacturing section of the firm. Consequently, it is central management which controls prices, the range of products, marketing, property costs, wages, and the inventory of the stores: and as the firms develop electronic point of sale data capture, so decisions about reordering and stock control will become increasingly automatic and centralised.

Within this centralised, hierarchical structure, store managers exercise no control over key commercial decisions, but they do 'own' their performance in a number of other respects. They continue to have considerable influence over the care and control of stock; they can decide on the mix of staff (part-time v full-time); they have no control over pay scales but they can use merit awards; they can decide whether to cut prices on special offers and how to react to changes in the local market or the weather. As one store manager commented: 'I use the weather forecast in planning stock levels – so in anticipation of hot weather I will put out lettuces and salad dressings'. And it is up to the store manager to meet customer standards on service and tradesmanship. A Supermarket director observed that 'Our concern is not just about the end result but about the way the manager does things, for we believe that outcomes will be affected by detail'; hence 'Retail is Detail' is an oft-repeated platitude. Thus a change of store manager, it is reckoned in HSR, can mean either a 5 per cent drop or improvement in performance.

Senior management recognises the importance of the individual manager and directs significant resources – both time and money – to the evaluation of the performance of individual stores. The emphasis is on the efficiency and effectiveness of store management – in other words, making the shop attractive to customers at a minimum cost –

rather than the day-to-day profitability of individual branches. The branches are indeed set financial targets but, in the words of one of the central managers, 'You can't just say, the return is OK – let's forget about it'. The significance of financial returns for individual stores is difficult to interpret for a number of reasons. First, the trade-off between long-term and short-term considerations: 'You might have policies which raise profits in the short term only' (we shall return to this point later). Second, the trade-off between short-term profits and long-term efforts to build up the reputation of the chain: 'High profits are not acceptable if there is also a high level of complaints'. Third, excellent profits may reflect a competitor closing down, while conversely the entry of a new competitor may cause a dip in profits.

So, both companies employ a similar range of quantitative and qualitative, financial and non-financial, performance indicators. At the centre a number of performance indicators are used to look at organisational performance. As one would expect, there is a set of financial indicators, including the profit-and-loss account, the volume and value of sales, and the 'return on capital'. But there is also a small range of non-financial indicators: for example, the percentage of orders that are met by the warehouse within a given time limit. At the periphery each organisation possesses a small set of key indicators. In HSR this is the monthly 'Three S' report which give figures for Staff, Sales, and Stock – with most emphasis being placed on the *ratio* between the three elements. In Supermarket there are about half a dozen core PIs which are used to evaluate the performance of individual stores.

However, this creates a paradox: despite the great and increasing emphasis on producing more performance-related data more quickly, there has also been a great and increasing emphasis in both organisations upon hands-on management: 'We are getting more information more quickly ... but it needs people to unravel it'. Indeed, HSR in particular uses the assessment of individual managers as a way of assessing the performance of stores. Here the emphasis is on 'understanding' the figures – i.e. the reasons for any given performance. In turn, this reflects the importance attached to taking a longer-term view and to taking into account the impact of the environment in which a branch operates: 'If you just look at the figures for one year, you might misjudge people because you don't know how much of the output is the product of the previous manager – a five year look allows you to disentangle the personal and store factors'. The philosophy here appears to be that if the key commercial decisions are taken at the centre, then the crucial element at the periphery is 'good' managers. And by 'good' the management means contented and motivated staff who are oriented to maximising customer satisfaction in a shop that is both clean and welcoming. In other words, performance assessment must focus on the *personal* performance and development of managers which are essential to achieve these aims. To satisfy this requirement, it has also been necessary to utilise a number of qualitative PIs to supplement the assessment of individual performance.

Each Supermarket branch calculates two key PIs – daily, weekly, monthly, etc. – using a strictly formalised set of procedures. First, the number of items put through the check-out divided by the available labour hours per hour – we shall call it Articles Per Hour (APH). Second, the APH actually achieved by a store divided by the standard it is expected to achieve – we shall call this the Performance Ratio (PR). In addition, Supermarket looks at the proportion of products available on the shelves each morning, the ratio of stocks against sales, and at the number of price reductions that a store has to make in order to sell its goods. These PIs are integrated into the daily/weekly reporting process of the Supermarket store manager. This provides detailed information which is available in an aggregated and disaggregated form to the directors: central managers have immediate access to the details of the performance of an individual store. Consequently, management is able to employ quite a sophisticated target-setting approach. Store managers are set normative standards for APH and PR by their area managers. These are calculated on a national basis, 'we can now go to a branch and say "our model predicts this for your branch" ', although a store may have individual features built into its figures – for example, by taking into account the opening of extra car parking space. A variety of performance checks can be made: the PR of an individual branch can be compared with that of branches of a similar size or location, or against the budgeted APH of a store. Although differences in store size make like-for-like comparisons difficult, nevertheless the fact that normative standards and ratios can reasonably be attributed to PIs does make these direct comparisons (and the inevitable resulting league tables) quite useful. However, it is interesting that even with the sophisticated Supermarket PI system, as with our public sector organisations, head-quarters tends to monitor 'by exception', picking up the outliers and ignoring the average performer.

This target-setting approach is also used in strategic planning when setting up new branches or in evaluating performance against that of competitors. When planning a new store, detailed estimates are made of expected performance figures in the first months of trading, and then re-adjusted until new standards are established for that store. Market share is another important indicator. The PIs are adapted by estimating the loss of trade following the opening of a new store by a competitor to reflect the re-adjustment of targets needed for the planned recovery of the supermarket store.

In contrast, HSR does not possess such detailed quantitative performance ratios. Consequently, its elaborate hierarchy of regional and area managers plays an important 'hands-on' role. They see themselves as 'travelling managers' aiming to spend as much as 80 per cent of their time on the road touring stores. At the beginning of every year, they agree on 'Three S' targets with each branch manager, and then every month 'every branch manager will be talked through his or her figures and will have to explain over or under performance'. The 'Three S' targets are transmitted hierarchically. Central management sets particular targets such as for sales. However, these are then negotiated for individual stores between the regional and branch managers. And they are seen as diagnostic tools as well as targets. If a branch manager fails to achieve his or her 'Three S' target, the regional or district manager will make frequent, unannounced visits.

But even if the 'Three S' targets are being achieved, it is not automatically assumed that the branch manager's performance is satisfactory: 'I would compare the performance with those of other, similar branches, both in my own area and elsewhere. Statistics don't tell you about the potential.' As in Supermarket, in comparing performance with that of other branches, the exercise would take account of both the characteristics of the stores themselves (space; design; lay-out) and environmental factors (major conurbation; market towns; seaside; rural). HSR also uses the Acorn system for categorising the local populations as a check on subjective hunches.

In assessing performance, there is much emphasis in both firms on running an efficient shop, in the sense of providing good customer service, i.e. service *is* the output. In contrast to the public sector, the key is that 'we have to attract customers'. Consequently, two negative, quantitative PIs are used to point out events or features that simply should not happen if the shop is being managed satisfactorily. First, both chains carry out regular sample checks on the availability of merchandise. Supermarket is particularly sophisticated in this respect because, by 9.30am daily, its directors receive details of a sample survey of stores recording the percentage of items not on the shelf that morning. Quite simply, the concern is to ensure that goods are actually on the shelves. Second, complaints are treated very seriously and regarded as a 'sensitive and important indicator'. Every HSR customer who complains is visited – usually within a week. In Supermarket, complaints are also closely monitored – both by store and by subject –

each one being individually scrutinised by a director: 'I take several home with me each night, although I leave it to the relevant department to write the reply'. In Supermarket, the number of complaints is small enough to make the subject area most important; as with the NHS 'the most popular grouse is always the length of the queues'!

It is interesting that the shelf-fill and complaint PIs are actually quantitative PIs of quality. Supermarket claims to take this concept further. Obviously there are additional checks on quality made by hygiene and safety inspectors. But, in addition, managers claim that 'Anything that isn't up to scratch can be detected somewhere in the figures'. In other words, if the APH and the performance ratios for a store are squeezed, then this will result in a slight lowering of customer standards. By relaxing the pressure a little, this will release staff time to improve quality. In this respect, Supermarket managers apply two standards: 'The "customer standard" ensures that all the items are on the shelves; the "Supermarket standard" is higher – the baked beans are all nicely piled up with their labels showing i.e. a good visual standard'.

Both organisations also attribute considerable importance to subjective judgement: 'A good area manager will be able to see when walking into a shop ... standards will be reflected in the general atmosphere and morale ... The manager will be able to sense it'. And, 'when you go into a store, you can feel it and see it'. Trying to put some flesh on this 'feeling', managers say that they will take into account the lengths of queues, the speed at which customers are served, and whether supervisors are around, but clearly it is based on years of managerial training and experience. Despite the active tradition whereby Supermarket directors make weekly visits to check-up on stores – 'tactile performance monitoring' – the emphasis on qualitative hands-on management is stronger in HSR, possibly because it has not yet devised a system of PIs that is as sophisticated as Supermarket's. In HSR – perhaps even more than in Supermarket where personnel managers do talk about customer service, about seeing that staff smile at customers, and so on – the key to performance and customer satisfaction is seen to lie in the way branch managers handle their own staff. This is the element in which branch managers have the largest degree of autonomy; i.e. in the management of people. They are free, for example, to increase staff cost if they also increase sales – since 'they are working a ratio'. To some extent this can be measured quantitatively by monitoring turnover and absenteeism figures: 'When you have a disciplined, well-run store, you get low absence and wastage rates'. Absenteeism is of growing interest in both firms because technology now makes it easier to distinguish between absence for holidays, training, and sickness. But again, management in HSR tends to stress intangible elements: 'The attitude of the staff is the most clear indicator of whether or not a store is being well managed'. In all this, 'figures only give you the clue – the signal to get in your car and have a look'.

Staff management and morale are thus seen as the key to good performance at the level of the individual branch; so performance is judged very much in terms of managerial *style*. As one regional manager put it 'I supplement the "Three S" targets with my own "Three Fs" criteria – firmness, fairness, and the ability to create a friendly environment'. Conversely, in a poorly run store 'you are likely to find that the manager is autocratic and withdrawn, with no involvement with either his or her own staff or customers'.

One last point. Amongst all our organisations, Supermarket stands out for the speed with which it generates PIs and makes them available for monitoring. Each store has a daily report which includes the key PIs and items like shelf-fill which is telephoned in to central office, so that each morning information about individual shops is available to the central managers. Although action at headquarters is normally left to weekly management meetings, where trends are analysed and policy discussed, it is possible for senior management to be quickly aware of problems and to make an immediate response. Of course, such extreme sensitivity may also reflect, apart from investment in new technology, the competitiveness of the food market and the perishable and variable nature of the product – shelf-life is less of an issue for a pullover or a book than it is for strawberries.

In summary, both Supermarket and HSR make significant use of non-financial PIs – both quantitative and qualitative – by integrating them into a process of branch evaluation that includes specific target-setting as well as the more subjective hands-on management. It is useful to highlight some of the (interesting) features that characterise the two PI systems.

The aim of the PI system as a whole is to deal with the problem of interdependence by identifying with precision the contribution of individual parts of the organisation (manufacturing, buying, delivery, retail). The objective is that if things go wrong there is no doubt about who owns the 'bad' performance. To monitor and control the performance of individual branches both systems concentrate on a small core of indicators that monitor the key aspects of managing an efficient organisation. Although modern information systems generate a large amount of information, the headquarters of Supermarket and HSR, unlike those in the NHS or the police, are not awash with statistics (often of peripheral importance). Where possible, quantitative PIs are used prescriptively to set targets based on explicitly normative standards. This is particularly so in Supermarket which boasts a system sophisticated enough to allow the management to apply numerical standards to measure at least some aspects of efficiency, effectiveness, and quality of customer service. One further feature of this system – which also explains the small number of PIs and their accuracy – is that the system is concept-driven, not data-driven. In other words, when designing this system, senior management knew precisely what they needed to measure in order to monitor performance; there was no need for superfluous PIs.

Both organisations also make use of negative PIs such as shelf-fill and complaints. These are used more descriptively (although senior management still applies normative standards about 'acceptable' levels) but are regarded as useful indicators of consumer access, choice, speed of performance, and quality. As such, they fit comfortably into the 'hands-on' style of management that characterises both organisations. Even in Supermarket, despite the relative sophistication of its concept-driven system of PIs, based as it is on a number of normative standards, much of the information gathered raises questions and still requires considerable interpretation.

Nevertheless HSR seems to be somewhat different from even our other private sector organisations in the emphasis put on branch performance, seen as the ability to pull in the customers. In short, while central management is responsible for the goods sold (their price and quality), it is branch management which is responsible for the quality of the *service*: the style and atmosphere in which the goods are sold. Although great importance is attributed to keeping the shelves filled, on displaying the goods well, on minimising losses due to pilfering and so on, HSR also (perhaps more than our other organisations) sees good performance in terms of the management of people rather than the management of goods.

MONEY-SHUFFLING IN THE HIGH STREET: BANK AND THE BUILDING SOCIETIES

The differences in the relative size of clearing banks and building societies may suggest that it is difficult to compare the two types of organisation. We can take size to refer to a number of dimensions: the number of branches, of employees, and the sheer scale of business. The traditional 'big four' clearing banks are much larger on all these criteria than even the largest building societies. Although both our building societies are in the top ten building societies – numbering several hundred branches (but excluding their 'agency' network) – this does not match the significantly larger branch network of Bank. Nevertheless it is our contention that Bank and Societies X and Z are comparable organisations in two important respects: one, they operate in a similar product market; two, their organisational structures, consisting of a large branch network under tight central control, bear a close resemblance. By understanding these common organisational features it is possible to appreciate the institutional context in which performance indicators have been developed in Bank, Society X, and Society Z.

First, there is a sizeable overlap in the business activities of banks and building societies. The deregulation of financial institutions during the 1980s coupled with a series of technological innovations produced a far more competitive market in which clearing banks and building societies compete across a wide range of 'personal business' products: mortgages, personal loans, insurance policies, cheque and deposit accounts and similar products and services. The main initiative for change came from the banks which discarded the traditional view of the UK banking system as a mechanism for recycling personal deposits into industrial loans; the new emphasis is on recycling personal deposits back to the personal sector as loans (*Lloyds Bank Economic Bulletin* 1988), no doubt because this is more profitable. Not surprisingly, competition has been particularly fierce in the home loans market where the clearing banks, with their large branch networks, were able to exercise a competitive advantage over the building societies in their traditional territory (ibid.). The banks have had considerable success: in 1980 the building societies had 82 per cent of home loans outstanding; by 1987 this had fallen to 72 per cent, with just 68 per cent of new loans.

The building societies have reacted strongly to this challenge. Most building societies remain wedded to their historical objective which is to attract savings which are then lent out in the form of home loans. While building societies have lost ground in the home loans market, they have successfully fended off bank incursions into the deposits market. Indeed, the banks' share of the market fell from 30 per cent to 26 per cent between 1980 and 1987, while the building societies increased their share from 54 per cent to 58 per cent over the same period (ibid.). Further, the building societies have fought back by offering their own interest-bearing cheque accounts and cash dispenser systems to challenge the previous monopoly of this product market by the banks. The building societies have also used their home loan base to build a strong insurance business. It is still true to say that banks are involved in wider markets which are either untouched by building societies or, like providing foreign currency and traveller's cheques, their stake in the market remains small. Nevertheless in terms of the business of the high street branch network, although banks still provide a broader range of products and services, there are important similarities in the basic functions of the individual branch.

Second, despite significant differences in legal form – clearing banks are public limited companies whereas building societies are registered as friendly societies under the Building Societies Act 1986 – the organisational structures and processes bear a close resemblance. Both are relatively low on heterogeneity and complexity. Over-simplifying only a little, clearing banks and building societies are organisations that are primarily concerned with money-shuffling. They provide a limited range of products, with little interdependence between different parts of the organisation, no marked variety in the skills required from staff, and, despite the need to acquire certain qualifications, no professionals. In all these respects, Bank and the building societies closely resemble Social Security.

The performance of the organisation, as a whole and for different branches, is highly dependent on the effectiveness of central policies involving the investment and use of acquired capital. Consequently, the degree of ownership of performance available to branch managers is limited. Interest rates are set nationally and the granting of loans is now largely determined by credit-scoring risk analysis rather than the personal discretion of the branch manager. In Bank, higher-risk commercial loans are normally hived off to specialist divisions. Marketing strategies are mainly dictated by central priorities and salaries are set nationally.

The performance of a branch may also be profoundly influenced by external factors. These may be largely outside the control of the organisation. For example, particularly in the case of Bank, the closure of a major commercial account can devastate the figures of a branch (although, of course, the decision to close may be as a result of poor service). Alternatively, there may be factors beyond the control of an individual branch manager. For example, Thomas (1982: 27) cites three key determinants of the performance of a branch; the office site, the immediate area in the vicinity of the branch, and its primary service or market area. He argues that all three of these locational factors should be favourable for an optimum site; put simply, 'it does matter where a facility is situated in or near a shopping centre, it does matter what side of the street it is on; and, it does matter what corner of an intersection it occupies' (ibid.: 27). Perhaps most important, and underlying all these locational factors, is the nature and degree of competition from other banks and building societies in the neighbourhood.

Given these similarities it seems reasonable to compare directly the three organisations in their approaches to performance measurement. In so doing, it should be noted that the analysis freely conflates all the organisations for much of the time because, quite simply, they offer a common experience.

Considering the limited scope that a branch manager has to influence profits, it may appear surprising that all three organisations have placed increasing emphasis on the development of indicators of branch performance. This policy is based on the firm belief that the quality of management is variable; as a director of one building society observed, 'there is a street-length difference between a good and a bad manager'. This said, the introduction of a formal branch evaluation programme is a quite recent phenomenon, not just in our case studies, but throughout the banking world (Thomas 1982). This is partly explained by the difficulties and costs of compiling the necessary database, prior to the advent of new information technology.

Branch evaluation takes two forms: financial and operational. There has always been some financial branch evaluation in which, like our retailers, the key indicators are profit and return on capital. Additional important ratios include branch profits against staff costs (a critical factor in a labour-intensive service organisation) and the absorption rate – a measure of running costs against branch income. These indicators provide a report on the performance of each location: branches failing to reach satisfactory returns on these financial measures are liable to come under close scrutiny. In Bank, all branches are ranked within their region. But calculating branch profit-and-loss is enormously complex, and ultimately quite subjective. How are the very large central costs of marketing and administration to be allocated to individual branches? What if different branches perform different primary functions? Thus in Society X there are two types of branch: feeder branches that deal with savings accounts and give advice on mortgages, and processing branches that handle all the mortgages from feeder branches as well as their own applications. The contrasting priorities given to functions by branches reflect different market locations: south coast retirement town branches will primarily attract investment money – while suburban branches will attract more applications for home loans. This makes individual profitability difficult to determine: the organisation needs both types of branch, but it is the mortgage-lending branch that actually makes the profits. So it is clear that the branch manager can exercise little direct influence over financial indicators.

Consequently, given the inappropriateness of judging branch

performance simply on the basis of financial PIs, each of our organisations has moved towards introducing branch evaluation programmes based on operational as opposed to financial indicators. This trend was strengthened by the need, in a rapidly changing market, to maintain a close scrutiny over short-term trends at branch level. Moreover, it is quite straightforward to develop non-profit performance indicators that monitor the operational areas over which a manager can exercise some control.

So what does a branch manager control? The main area is marketing; an answer that may confound the traditional stereotyped view of the boring, unimaginative bank manager. For the successful bank manager today is a person who excels at marketing services and products, rather than the generalist administrator who keeps a tidy branch. Even here the options open to the manager are closely tied into the central marketing strategy; if Bank is undertaking an expensive, high profile, national campaign to 'sell' more credit cards, then it is obviously in a branch manager's own interest to reap the benefits by pushing credit cards in her or his own branch. However, there is some scope to pursue local marketing strategies. For example, the south coast building society branch might advertise premium investment accounts to attract the savings of pensioners, while the city centre branch will seek to persuade wage-earners with the more flexible lower interest accounts. Similarly, the Bank branch in an affluent suburban area may push high interest cheque accounts, while a branch in a poor inner city area may emphasise personal loans. It is also worth noting that the successful manager will, to some extent, be a risk-taker: 'the manager who has no bad debts is a bad manager'. Thus the modern branch manager will face a conflict between the desire 'to keep your nose clean' and the need to take various risks and initiatives necessary to become a 'high flyer'.

The basic indicators measure the number of products issued – home loans, insurance policies, credit cards, high interest cheque accounts, cash dispenser cards, Eurocheque cards, etc. – and the value of services like home loans, personal loans, high interest accounts, insurance premiums, arrangement and lending fee income, etc. (it is important to monitor both volume and value as it is cheaper to make fewer, higher value loans because arrangement costs vary little with the size of the loan). Many of these examples are common to all three organisations, notably home loans and insurance premiums, but others, like credit cards, are confined to Bank. Furthermore, these general categories are usually disaggregated: for example, insurance premiums are divided into buildings, house contents, life, mortgage protection, repayment, and a host of additional policies such as travel insurance.

These indicators in themselves merely provide a descriptive picture of trends in branch performance which may raise questions, but without detailed knowledge of circumstances provide no definitive evaluation of performance. However, these PIs are incorporated into a branch evaluation report that regularly monitors managerial performance. The key feature of this report is a series of performance targets. In the past, the setting of targets involved a loosely controlled bottom-up system in which individual branch managers selected their own personal targets and simply reported them upwards. More recently, the achievement of operational targets has been given greater priority; just as the shop manager is expected to shift goods, so bank or building society managers are judged on their ability to shift financial services. Consequently, the process is, of necessity, more centralised and sophisticated: target-setting is a negotiated process in which the branch manager suggests targets that are adjusted by the district manager, who is the final arbiter.

The greater detail and objectivity underpinning the new approach is made possible by the increased quantity and reliability of information about the performance of the individual branch, the comparative performance of other branches in similar areas or of comparable size, and detailed knowledge of the local market based on customer profiles and existing market penetration. This enables the district and area managers to adopt a far more directive role in negotiations. One senior Bank manager explained 'If the manager of a branch that issued fifty credit cards last year says they will go for seventy this year, I may now say that a branch that size should be issuing 200 cards'. A Bank district manager commented that

> The negotiation of these targets is crucial. We have data going back over previous years to form a time-series which helps to set targets. I need to look for past under-achievers who may be getting an apparently large percentage increase yet they are starting from a very low base. This makes the penetration figure very important – I can't expect a 90 per cent credit card figure to improve very much!

This negotiation process also allows the district manager to advise branch managers about national priorities to ensure that the prime branch objectives are congruent with planned national marketing campaigns.

Nevertheless the targets are still essentially subjective, as is the use that management makes of them. Each district manager will closely monitor performance: scrutinising monthly figures and making quarterly visits to branches to discuss performance against targets. Questions are asked about missed targets, whether under- or over-achieving, in order to discover whether there is a valid external explanation or whether it is simply down to poor management. Some managers develop their own systems for interpreting performance against targets. One Bank district manager set forty-one targets, each rated on a scale of between one and four points: four points for priority objectives for that year such as home loans and high interest cheque accounts, dropping to just one point for deposit accounts. He then gave points for achievement: one point for 80–100 per cent, two for 101–150 per cent, three for 150–200 per cent, and four for anything over 200 per cent. Thus a 100 per cent accurate home loan figure received four points, a 250 per cent figure received sixteen points! The points were aggregated for all forty-one targets, enabling him to rank his thirty branches for overall performance.

There is a system of performance-related pay and profit sharing in the building societies in which the rewards for a positive personal appraisal are closely tied into the achievement of branch objectives. Bank is going along the same road, paying a small bonus to all the staff if the branch achieves its targets. As one senior Bank manager observed 'this bonus is not high, but the aim is to bring in some competition between branches in order to get individual branches to work as a team'. It is certainly implicit in the Bank evaluation system that it is the performance of the manager which is being evaluated, rather than that of the branch. However, unless the manager can motivate the staff to emphasise customer service and to push various services, he or she is unlikely to achieve agreed targets.

But the subjective nature of target-setting raises problems. A senior Bank manager admitted that 'last year, several branches exceeded targets but received no reward because other branches did even better'. More objective indicators like market penetration are available – 'if there are two branches with 5000 customers and one has sold 500 home loans, the other 1000 loans; why is one performing better?' – but while regional managers possess this detailed data for their own region, they only receive aggregate figures for other regions. Work is under way to develop the means of directly comparing like-with-like, such as all market town branches, but at present the three organisations only have rankings within a region. One regional manager in Society X reflected

> We are moving towards individual profit management. We are advised about the profit of the area but we are not yet targeted on it because of the problems of measurement. Whether it will be based on individual branches, or clusters, or areas – time will tell.

But how can individual circumstances be acknowledged? For example, the classic case, mentioned in each of our organisations, of the 'clean-up job' appointment – the manager who is sent in to clear up the mess created by previous poor management. Here growth is clearly not the short-term objective, but how will this be recognised in a set of comparative figures?

It is worth emphasising that each organisation stresses the importance of regarding the performance review process 'not as a snapshot, but as a constant dialogue; a regular, open, dialogue that seeks to identify problems and weaknesses rather than impose sanctions', as a director of Society Z put it. There are also a number of staff-centred, non-profit indicators. Although salaries and establishments are set centrally, there is some flexibility open to management, and, as staffing accounts for around 70 per cent of overall costs in all three organisations, any savings here will be important.

First, productivity; as one manager commented 'every cashier will tell me that he or she has been busy, so we need to measure it'. However, although it is a relatively straightforward task to measure the volume of transactions in order to set the establishment level (and subsequently to monitor it), this procedure raises serious problems of case-mix. Thus the south coast branch may be quite relaxed except on Thursdays – pension day – when staff are overstretched and need longer per customer. Or the mortgage interview for the first-time buyer will take longer than for old hands. These are all familiar case-mix issues which make it imperative that the quantitative indicator is not treated as a definitive measure. Second, absenteeism is regularly monitored. Third, continually high levels of overtime may indicate that a manager is asking staff to do too much overtime to protect individual branch profit levels. Fourth, staff turnover; but this is closely tied up with the local labour market – the number of available jobs and comparative wage levels. Ironically, if staff turnover is too high, then it might be in the interests of the branch to provide regular overtime to dissuade staff from leaving.

As in many other organisations, the key to the recent introduction of the more sophisticated branch evaluation system is the availability of improved information systems based on new technology. All three of our financial organisations have an information system that serves different purposes at each level. The central office is only really concerned with aggregated figures which provide an overview of, say, the national and regional performance on home loans. In contrast, at local level the disaggregated data have allowed area and regional managers to monitor branch performance more closely. But, in essence, as the director of Society Z observed, 'what started as an improved information base has become a control base'. Even if the centre is not exercising direct control with disaggregated data, it is exercising indirect control through regional and area management structures.

Yet the distance of the central office from the performance of the branches – the disaggregated data from the individual Bank branch will not even be passed on to the centre – contrasts sharply with, for example, the 'hands-on' approach of Supermarket where directors closely scrutinise such data and make frequent personal visits to stores. One explanation for this is the smaller number of shops compared with bank branches; thus the building societies (with fewer branches and fewer services) seem to monitor performance a little more closely than Bank. But it also reflects a contrasting management style between the 'retail is detail' hands-on approach of the retailers, and the more distant approach of the financial institutions.

Nevertheless the financial institutions can no longer afford to take their customers for granted; since deregulation the increasingly competitive market has forced them to focus on the standard of service they provide to the customer. One traditional instrument of quality control is the inspectorate which visits branches every two to three years. In Bank the formal visit of the inspectorate still involves a comprehensive examination of virtually every item, whereas the building societies' inspectorate adopts a slightly more relaxed approach. Although the main functions of the inspectorate are audit (the National Westminster Bank estimates that mistakes by employees account for 25–40 per cent of the total costs of any service business [*The Economist*, 15 July 1989]) and to maintain security, it inevitably scrutinises the performance of tasks from a quality angle. Put simply, are tasks being carried out according to correct procedures? In addition, as one Society X regional manager commented, 'the inspectors' report is a useful guide for me because they actually see the manager in action, at the sharp end – though rarely do I get an opinion conflicting with my own assessment'.

However, there are few specific quality PIs in any of the three organisations, largely because it appears to be difficult to devise such measures. There are one or two quantitative measures that assess the quality of managerial decisions: for example, it is regarded as dangerous to have too many 100 per cent mortgages; better to have a balance that includes a number of 50 per cent loans. But the most frequent quality indicator is the familiar, instinctive one; as one senior Bank manager put it 'You just know whether the branch provides a quality service to customers', and, similarly, a Society Z manager remarked 'you can smell a well-run office'. Each organisation stresses the importance of the customer, and each is firmly committed to various types of total quality management influenced 'customer care' or 'customer first' programmes.

Thus Society X stresses the importance of 'people', whether initiating a new openness with staff and ploughing resources into staff training, or with customers, by actively encouraging them to make complaints. A regional manager in Society X sums up the new philosophy: 'the variety and number of complaints is now increasing but we are changing our response – we will now be more honest in our response so that we can get away from seeing the complaint as a negative thing but as something we can learn from'.

But do customers approve of these changes and do they find it easy to make a complaint? The answer to this as yet thinly researched question may be uncovered by the various customer surveys, for which there is a new-found enthusiasm across the financial sector (Buswell 1986). The impact of this philosophy must be open to question, for while both building societies do monitor the number and type of complaints at all levels, at least in Society Z it is all rather low key: 'it is a barometer check but not very reliable . . . it is not a primary performance indicator'. Perhaps more important than the sheer quantity of complaints is the level at which they surface. For although the organisations have a formal complaints procedure where area managers are responsible for resolving and responding to problems, it is acknowledged in Bank and Society X that if a complaint reaches senior management level then this will prompt a speedier, higher level reaction. But high level involvement is not routinised. Clearly the banks have a long way to go before they adopt the approach of Famibank (a Belgian subsidiary of Citibank) which monitors the number of telephone calls it takes to solve a customer's problem and the number of times a customer is bounced from counter to counter before a query is resolved (*The Economist*, 15 July 1989). This kind of disaggregated, quantitative monitoring, on the lines of Supermarket, could be adopted in Social Security as easily as it could be in the financial institutions.

It has already been noted that the PIs of each organisation are reported at a rather leisurely pace. Roughly, the common pattern involves the district manager getting monthly figures from branches and making quarterly visits to monitor progress directly against the branch plan. Higher up, the aggregated regional performance is monitored monthly against plans. All three organisations seem to lack the capacity to make the instant response to operational problems that is contained in Supermarket's system.

This difference is probably largely explained by the historical inertia that characterises the product market. This is most apparent in banking, where, traditionally, there has been a high level of customer loyalty; most people stay with the same bank all their lives, often the one that their parents banked with, and the vast majority of customers visit their branch less than once a year (a further factor reducing the scope of a manager to affect performance). The scenario may be slightly less static in building societies but the profile looks similar. Certainly, although the market is becoming more competitive, if people do move their accounts it is still usually for the negative reason that they have received poor service, rather than the positive attraction of a competitor.

Nevertheless the slow reporting of PIs and the low emphasis on using quality PIs also suggest a lower sensitivity to the customer than in, say, Supermarket. Quite simply, Bank does not need to be as customer-sensitive because its biggest profits (or losses) are made in the money markets, and its customers will remain loyal unless the branch does something stupid. This said, with the market becoming more competitive, even Bank is having to become more aware of customer needs. Indeed, the introduction of the PI system is itself a manifestation of this changing market. None of our organisations can afford to have poor performing branches.

SERVICING THE CUSTOMER: JUPITER TVHIRE

Jupiter is a large company with several different businesses, one of which is TVhire. TVhire itself has two separate businesses: television rentals (with a small sales side) and television servicing. On both sides of the organisation there is a large chain of shops – several hundred rental outlets but less than one hundred service centres. Like our retailers, each shop must prove that it is profitable. However, the nature of the relationship with the customer is quite different from the normal retailer because the contract to hire a television creates an ongoing agreement and a continuous relationship with the customers.

It is relatively simple to establish performance criteria for the shops because there is a reasonably clear bottom line to form the basis of a profit-and-loss account. However, in the service business there is no income bottom line – work is carried out as part of the rental contract – so the performance criterion is whether an individual branch is maximising efficiency in the use of resources. The issue is further complicated by the link between rentals and service. If customers receive poor service then this may cause the number of rentals to decline, but this will only show up in the performance indicator system when the damage has been done. Nonetheless it is a relevant consideration because, as one senior manager confessed, 'if we are missing targets in one year then we would meet them by fiddling cash which would mean hitting service, which in time will hit the rentals side!'

So the measurement of shop performance is straightforward. Apart from simple financial measures such as the level of income and of costs, there are a number of non-financial performance indicators. Given that the main yardsticks for success involve 'the ability to obtain a customer contract and then to hang on to it', the PIs measure the number of new agreements, the number of 'ceasehires' – customers terminating their agreement – and the ratio of the volume of ceasehires against new agreements. The importance of these measures is obvious in that they have a direct bearing on the future performance of the company; as one manager commented 'it is an issue of stocks and flows'.

In contrast, without any direct income, it is difficult to construct financial indicators on the service side, except simple cost measures such as the consumption of materials. So the company monitors an array of indicators: notably, the proportion of new rentals installed within forty-eight hours, the number of service calls cleared within twenty-four hours, the number of technicians per subscriber, the average length of time of a service visit, and the number of ceasehires and of complaints (an approach that, as we shall see, is rather similar to the water industry). Indeed, the validity of these PIs is all the more important on the service side because its cost structure is potentially quite variable, whereas shop costs are relatively fixed.

These indicators are built into a time-series and used as the basis for annual target-setting. Target-setting is a negotiated process, albeit with the balance of power heavily in favour of senior management. But managers have to be very careful because 'the agreed targets are expected to take the environment, inflation, and so on into account so that managers own their performance'. All the key PIs feed into a bonus scheme. This scheme has a numerical scale with the target as a median point; branch performance will be rewarded according to the point that a manager achieves on the scale. However, central management makes a subjective judgement on the level of the bonuses, informed by years of experience about what is an achievable target.

Three further points are worth mentioning. First, TVhire provides another example of senior management dealing only in aggregated figures: 'It is the responsibility of the next level down to provide detail; detail is a check, the currency of explanation, the managers need to know the detail to run the company. We can't know the detail of each company.' From the point of view of central management 'We control the big numbers and if the big numbers go wrong I can call the manager in charge to account. It is about a critical mass.' Second, nevertheless, central management recognizes the importance of timeliness by ensuring that key indicators like the volatile retail sales figures are available each Monday, or even the next day, for scrutiny. Where speed is less important, as on the rental side which is a more stable business, the indicators form the basis of a monthly performance review. Third, TVhire applies its PIs to its outlets in other countries: 'we assume a logic but not a consistency in PIs across countries. If the nature of the business is the same then PIs should be the same. Managers must provide explanation for variation.'

SUMMARY

It is quite clear then that the use of non-profit performance indicators is playing an increasingly important role in organisations right across the private sector. Managers in each of the organisations discussed in this chapter have found it difficult to isolate the performance of individual branches. Certainly they draw up a profit-and-loss account for each branch and make frequent use of financial indicators, such as return on capital and costings, but it is recognized that these do not provide a complete or even accurate picture of branch performance. One solution to this problem is the development of operational performance indicators that measure aspects of performance for which a branch manager can be held responsible.

In themselves, these non-financial indicators – the number of items passing through a shop check-out each hour, the number of new credit cards issued, the average time taken to service a television – merely provide a descriptive account of what a branch has done. But by building these indicators into an annual target-setting process, with regular monitoring of performance against those targets, they can be transformed into an effective instrument of central management control over branch activity. Thus descriptive indicators are given a prescriptive role. There are quantitative and qualitative indicators, and there are several negative indicators that point out things that simply should not happen in a well-run organisation – empty shelves, complaints, or staff absenteeism. Possibly of greatest significance is the general preference for parsimony; each organisation has adopted a small core of indicators – roughly between six and ten in total – with the merits of clarity, simplicity, and accessibility; features not obviously prevalent in the public sector. Thus profit may provide the motor for the development of PIs in the private sector but the PIs themselves often have nothing to do with money.

6 Managing monopolies
Railways, water, and airports

This chapter examines the development of performance indicators in three organisations: British Rail, the Water Authorities, and BAA (formerly the British Airports Authority). They share a number of features in common, most notably for our purposes a long-standing and continuing interest in the development of performance indicators. Indeed, this interest has produced three sets of organisational performance indicators that are generally more sophisticated in design and attractive to use than other public sector systems. Yet it is important to point out that each organisation developed its system of performance evaluation while in public ownership, although subsequently BAA was privatised in 1987 and the water authorities were sold off in November 1989.

As with all nationalised industries, each organisation has had to grapple with the problem of hands-off ministerial control: in short, how can a commercial organisation remain accountable to Parliament without unnecessary interference in the day-to-day management of the business? The problem was highlighted in the report of the first Select Committee on Nationalised Industries in 1968:

> The fact that Ministerial responsibility for the efficiency of the industries is at one step removed makes it the more necessary that Ministers should have criteria by which to judge them. They must lay down standards against which performance can be objectively measured, and provide themselves with feedback for the purpose of making these measurements.
>
> (Select Committee (1968), para. 73)

And later on:

> ... the figures at the bottom of the accounts – the accountant's profit

or loss – are not necessarily indicative of an industry's efficiency: Ministerial interventions on prices, monopoly powers, external factors such as interest rates or social obligations and other factors may distort the picture. Nor is a subjective judgment of the value of the industry's contributions to the nation likely to be a more reliable test. What is needed is some indication of the efficiency of the industry in performing both the commercial and the social duties that have been given to them by statute or by Ministers.

(ibid.: para. 155)

However, although the interest in PIs, at least in financial indicators, goes back a long way, with the exception of British Rail, these early exhortations had only limited impact.

A more important catalyst for change in all three organisations was the Labour Government's White Paper on Nationalised Industries in 1978 which called specifically for the production and publication of 'a number of key performance indicators' – including PIs for standards of service and productivity – and 'to make public suitable aims in terms of performance and service' (para. 78). The observable response of nationalised industries to these recommendations was to publish far more financial and non-financial performance data in annual reports and accounts, although the overall amount of available information remained limited (Mayston 1985; Woodward 1986). The pressure to generate financial PIs was increased by the Conservative Government's decision to impose strict 'external financial limits' on every nationalised industry, preventing access to public funds (although again it was the 1974–9 Labour Government that had introduced external limits).

What is of particular interest is that despite the denationalisation of these two organisations, all of them continue to be subject to public accountability because of the need to control public service monopolies. Each of these organisations can be classified as a monopoly. As we shall see, the monopoly position of water and BAA is self-evident; neither faces any competition in the market place. British Rail is in a slightly different position; obviously it possesses a monopoly over the railways but it is only one actor within the broader transport sector. However, it does have a large number of captive consumers, notably commuters, and it remains, for the present, in public ownership. So, although another shared feature is that they are all trading organisations, each with a 'bottom line' (like private firms), there remains, nevertheless, the extra dimension of accountability: all three organisations combine public accountability with involvement in market transactions.

Thus a number of factors have prompted each of the three organisations studied in this chapter to direct considerable effort and resources to developing PIs; if only for the symbolic purposes of satisfying the Government. This chapter examines the nature of these PIs and the extent to which they are actually being used within these organisations.

BRITISH RAIL

British Rail (BR) is one of the few remaining nationalised industries, although the Conservative Government has made clear its intention to privatise it. BR is very much in the public eye. It is politically accountable through its 'arm's-length' relationship with Government and Parliament, and is subject to a particularly close scrutiny from parliamentary questions, select committees, the Monopolies and Mergers Commission, and its official consumer watchdog, the Central Transport Consultative Committee (CTCC) and its regional committees. Network SouthEast commuters angered by cancelled trains or InterCity travellers inconvenienced by having to stand for long distances have plenty of outlets for their complaints.

BR is a large employer: in March 1988 there were 133,567 staff working on the railways (although the Board employed 154,748 staff including all its subsidiary businesses). It also boasts a rather complicated organisational structure. Traditionally BR's structure has been a combination of geographical and functional management. The headquarters conceive the strategy, and the six regions, composed of the regional, divisional (removed in 1984), and area tiers, run the railways. Five business sectors – Network SouthEast, InterCity, Provincial (divided into three subsidiary businesses: Express, Rural, and Urban), Freight, and Parcels – were introduced in 1982 at headquarters level thereby forming a three-dimensional organisational matrix (although as this book went to press, another reorganisation of sectors was under way). The intention is that areas report to the region for budgetary and functional purposes but that the sectors are allocated all the capital resources and have 'bottom-line' responsibility. Thus the responsibilities and activities of the sectors overlap with those of the area. To complicate matters further, some freight areas report directly to the Freight Sector on 'business matters'. Lastly, a number of separate functions, such as personnel, have been formed at headquarters with their own support staff. This rather clumsy structure at BR headquarters inevitably results in some confusion in the lines of authority over the sectors and the regional organisation.

This organisational structure reflects not so much a heterogeneity of products as the sheer complexity of operating a large railway network. It is not a complexity resulting from mixing and matching a broad collection of skills, as in the NHS; BR has a vast 'invisible' workforce that possesses little worker autonomy, despite the traditional pride associated with certain jobs such as that of train driver. Rather the complexity arises from the enormous degree of interdependence that is inherent in planning and operating the railways. Punctuality is the aspect of performance that raises the most manifest problems; one glance at the intricacies of a BR timetabling plan immediately conveys this point. The familiar platform announcement that a train is running late may have extensive implications for dozens of other trains, resulting in late departures, missed connections, and hence poor performance indicators. By way of contrast, it is interesting to note that one of BR's competitors, British Airways, unlike BR, only measures departure times and does not even attempt to measure arrival times because they are regarded as being beyond the control of the organisation.

Although possessing an almost complete monopoly over the railways, BR has to operate in a highly competitive transport industry alongside private cars, buses, coaches, road freight, London Transport, and airlines to name only the leading characters. Moreover, unlike most of its competitors BR cannot compete on purely commercial terms. Governments use nationalised industries to achieve a variety of political goals, from controlling inflation by holding down prices and wages, to reflating the economy through large capital projects. These objectives are liable to change at short notice. In common with other nationalised industries, BR was long instructed to aim for commercial viability at least in the InterCity, Freight, and Parcel sectors, but it was not until 1983–4 that the Thatcher Government specified clear targets and time-scales, i.e. strict external financial limits and the achievement of a 2.7 per cent return on net assets employed before interest by 1989–90 for these three sectors (BRB 1988). BR also has various social obligations, which are partially subsidised by the Public Service Obligation (PSO) grant – a subsidy introduced by the government to help relieve road congestion (particularly on Network SouthEast) and to help maintain uneconomic rail services for certain communities (CTCC 1989: 9). But the PSO subsidy was substantially reduced by 35 per cent between 1982 and 1988 (Pendleton 1988).

In other words, BR faces some uncertainty because it is constantly struggling to balance its multiple, ever-changing, commercial and social objectives. Should it seek long-term profit maximisation, the achievement of external financial limits, the provision of a quality rail service, or the maintenance of uneconomic railway lines? Clearly, these objectives are incompatible: each year the annual report proclaims success in the reduction of jobs and costs; each year the Central Transport Consultative Committee (CTCC), the official rail-users' 'watchdog', bemoans the priority given to short-term financial objectives at the apparent expense of the social objectives of quality and provision of service, as one might expect. In other respects, BR performance is rather lower on uncertainty; in operational terms, the relationship between inputs, outputs, and outcomes appears straightforward, barring the uncertainty resulting from environmental factors such as inclement weather conditions or vandalism of tracks and trains.

Undoubtedly the most powerful and persuasive pressure during the 1980s was to achieve government financial and productivity targets. This forced the BR Board to intensify its long-term strategy of cost-reduction rather than revenue-maximisation: the emphasis was on staffing reductions, lowering unit costs, raising productivity, and improving the utilisation of rolling stock. Although there has been a long-term contraction in the size of the workforce – the large fall of 14 per cent since the end of 1983 (BRB 1988) continues a decline in staffing that dates back to the 1950s and was particularly acute in the Beeching era (Pendleton 1988) – the recent rationalisation resulted from a determined effort by BR management to improve productivity throughout the organisation. It is in this context of a business dominated by considerations of cost-cutting that BR developed its PIs.

The design and use of performance indicators in British Rail

Amongst all our organisations, British Rail has one of the longest histories of introducing top-down performance measurement. In the 1950s BR was using rather crude physical indicators combined with a few financial indicators such as 'cost per parcel handled'. The choice of these PIs was largely accidental, based on statistics that originated in the plethora of forms that characterised the bureaucratic ethos of the organisation during that period. The business was said to be 'production-led'; it was the local chief of operations who decided which of these PIs to use and which were relevant; i.e. they were top-down in origin but they were often used quite differently at each local level. By the late 1950s with the dominance of work study and similar ideas, managers recalled that 'if it moved, it got measured'. By tying the indicators into the bonus scheme the system grew even more complex and bureaucratic. With the onset of the Beeching review and resulting cuts in the early 1960s, there was a move to financial management which saw the demise of BR's old army-style management. Budgets became the goal; every level and function had budgets to measure performance (indeed, despite the subsequent efforts of reformers within BR, budgets still remain dominant).

The next change occurred after the 1978 White Paper and the Conservative victory of 1979 which increased the pressure on BR to improve productivity. The 'Productivity Steering Group' was set up at headquarters level; an internal mission document, *Challenge of the 80s*, was produced in 1979; and a productivity deal was negotiated as part of the 1980 pay agreement. The intention was to achieve significant productivity improvements through rationalisation and the removal of a planned 6000 posts.

As part of this initiative, BR developed its first reasonably comprehensive set of PIs. The Productivity Steering Group developed what was effectively a total system for the whole organisation, consisting of some 244 performance indicators. Within this system a hierarchy operated: every production department had PIs and each senior manager had about six PIs which increased at each level downwards so that at the disaggregated bottom line level all 244 indicators were in operation. There were many input and output measures, with outputs being measured against financial or physical criteria. Thus for passenger services, inputs were staffing and service costs, and outputs were measured either in terms of receipts or the number of train miles. Thus efficiency PIs could be constructed that related, for example, output measured in terms of train miles to sales volumes: so passenger service PIs included 'passenger train service costs per loaded train mile' and 'passenger receipts per loaded train mile'.

However, as all area managers were now held responsible for agreed targets there was considerable debate about whether these particular PIs were appropriate; many local and line managers complained bitterly that the PIs used to judge their performance were simply not relevant. Consequently a core of thirty-six PIs was agreed that covered every aspect of productivity although local managers were allowed to select those relevant to their own activities: a parcels manager, for example, would use the relevant PI in order to compare performance with other areas but if there was no parcels section locally then this PI would simply not be used. This encouraged the area managers to concentrate on the key thirty-six indicators.

The objectives of the PI system were twofold. One was to control management performance: 'Managers who are responsible for achievement are being clearly identified and made accountable; also a major development is the use of performance indicators for the first time to set budget targets' (BRB 1981). However, this was very much a 'first attempt' at measurement. What undermined its impact was the absence of any common standards or yardsticks against which to compare performance: 'the trouble was that a manager could only be held responsible for what had been individually agreed for that manager, so there was no question of drawing up valid league tables'. Consequently, in practice, according to one senior manager, the PIs were often used inconsistently and arbitrarily: 'we had problems with "baronial" managers taking the PIs and going off to use them to kick bottoms'. Thus the use of PIs in the control budget was simply to ensure that performance levels 'maintained or bettered previous best values'. Second, PIs were used in an effort to obtain genuine productivity improvement through 'best practice' by comparison both with objectives and through some attempt to produce tables not for personal accountability but to investigate significant variation in performance within the organisation.

The emphasis of the PI system was on describing performance; PIs were essentially tin-openers. Where PIs were used to manage specific changes at a local level their value was, inevitably, finite. And the PIs were predominantly concerned with efficiency. Very few PIs monitored the quality of service; punctuality and cancellation PIs were given little prominence in internal documents like the 1982 *Productivity Performance* report or in planning and budgeting processes.

Further developments in the use of PIs during the 1980s sprang from major changes in corporate strategy. This was partly the result of external political pressure. In the early years of the Thatcher Administration, BR had seemingly placated the Government by using a plethora of crude PIs to report apparent 'improvements' in productivity. But the Government became impatient with the way poor information about the performance of BR effectively obstructed the setting and monitoring of targets (Ferner 1988). An example of a crude use of PIs was the BR claim, made throughout the 1980s, that 'staff productivity, expressed as train miles per member of staff' was improving. Yet this PI took no account of rising overtime which probably absorbed most of the apparent improvement.

With the decision by the Government to adopt tougher financial limits and targets, BR could no longer hide behind the symbolic protection of favourable PIs. Apart from the more obvious manifestation of this change in attitude, namely the 'macho management' that provoked the flexible rostering dispute of 1982 (Ferner 1988; Pendleton 1988), a series of management reviews identified a number of areas where productivity and effectiveness could be improved. This resulted in the introduction of a new planning process in 1983, the integration of planning and budgeting outcomes, the publication of a ten year plan to improve productivity, and the establishment of firm action plans throughout the organisation, all of which combined to give a new significance to PIs. In particular, the corporate plans now included PIs as a means of measuring performance against specific internal financial targets and quality of service objectives drawn up the BR Board. As a result, rather than forming a separate, almost academic list containing hundreds of statistics, the PI package was streamlined and better integrated into the actual business management of BR. In other words, there was a transition from the development of a system of measurement, to a process of measuring how BR was actually performing and the integration of these PIs into management systems. In the words of one manager, 'we had left the question of analysis and we were now concerned with doing something about it'.

Recent annual reports contain some fifty-four PIs for the five core BR businesses; however, this includes those PIs disaggregated for the five businesses (see Table 6.1). This listing confirms the continued emphasis on cost-reduction and productivity – the total includes just ten quality of service PIs. Nevertheless a growing emphasis is being put, albeit slowly, on quality of service objectives. A number of factors account for this. Politically, the quality of service has come under increasing scrutiny from politicians and public. The Public Accounts Committee (1986) argued that the reduction of the Public Service Obligation grant meant that it was even more important to monitor quality of service and recommended that the Department of Transport should agree service objectives with the BR Board. The following year the Secretary of State formally agreed quality of service objectives for Network SouthEast for the first time and, following an MMC (1989) report on passenger services provided by the Provincial sector, new service quality objectives were set for this sector in 1989. But InterCity still has no formal requirements. Quality of service objectives are now included in the corporate plans (see Table 6.2). These objectives – for punctuality, queueing at ticket offices, train enquiry bureaux, cancellations, carriage cleaning, and load factors – are agreed for all the businesses. 'We used to complain that quality is ignored but we are now far more aware of quality targets', although some managers still bemoan the unfairness of being judged by PIs that are influenced by factors beyond their control.

Network SouthEast receives particular attention from politicians because it is a highly subsidised, heavily used commuter service which has suffered from serious problems of overcrowding and cancellations.

Table 6.1 British Rail performance indicators: a selection showing the performance of the total business and of the InterCity sector

	1984–5	1985–6	1986–7	1987–8	1988–9
Total rail business					
Total receipts per train mile (£)	9.23	9.34	9.48	9.52	9.47
Total operating expenses per train mile (£)	13.83	13.42	12.85	12.58	11.54
Train miles per member of staff (total staff productivity)	1726	1774	1812	1967	2123
Revenue per £1000 gross paybill costs (£)	1430	1479	1510	1594	1711
Train miles per train crew member (train crew productivity)	8045	8252	8564	9568	10485
Train miles per single track mile (000)	12.4	12.5	12.6	13.1	13.5
InterCity business					
Profit/loss as a percentage of receipts (£)	(3.0)	(21.1)	(16.0)	(12.4)	0.7
Receipts per train mile (£)	11.53	12.73	13.50	14.31	14.60
Receipts per passenger mile (£)	7.73	8.15	8.43	8.44	8.72
Passenger miles per loaded train mile (average train load)	155	161	165	175	174
Total operating expenses per train mile (£)	16.47	15.64	15.89	16.28	13.61
Percentage of trains arriving within ten minutes of booked time	n/a	n/a	85	87	87
Percentage of trains cancelled	n/a	n/a	0.8	0.5	1.0

Source: British Railways Board (1989) *Annual Report and Accounts 1988/89*

A Monopolies and Mergers Commission (MMC) report (1987) offered several recommendations to improve quality of service on Network SouthEast, paying particular attention to load factors. BR initially only produced a loading figure for Network SouthEast, but accepted the MMC (1989) recommendation to 'set, publish, and monitor load factor standards' for the Provincial sector. But BR produces an average figure for the entire business which is quite unhelpful and begs questions about the setting of standards. Both the MMC and the CTCC argue that to have any meaning this average must be broken down on a line by line basis, otherwise the existence of grossly overcrowded services is

Table 6.2 Rail passenger quality of service objectives – 1987

	InterCity	*NSE*	*Provincial*
Punctuality	On time and up to 10 mins late 90%	On time and up to 5 mins late 90%	On time and up to 5 mins late 85–97%
Service provision (% of services to run)	at least 99.5%	at least 99%	at least 98.5%
Carriage cleaning:			
– interior daily clean	100%	100%	95–100%
– external daily wash	95%	100%	75–100%
– heavy interior (per 28 days)	95%	100%	90–100%
Train enquiry bureaux	95% of calls to be answered within 30 seconds		
Ticket offices	Maximum queueing time of 5 mins peak and 3 min off-peak		
Load factors	–	No more than 135% for sliding door stock or 110% for slam door stock. No forced standing for over 20 minutes	

Source: British Railways Board (1987) *Corporate Plan*: 30–1.

disguised. The CTCC (1988) argues that 'when the existing load factor standards were originally agreed ... it was clearly understood that the figures of 110% and 135% [see Table 6.2] were maximum loadings for individual trains, not average targets to be aimed at and against which timetables are planned' (11). Moreover, the targets relate to *planned* train formations; they do not take account of the daily reductions in train size that push up load levels.

PIs are used both at different levels and for a variety of purposes within BR; a good example of this is punctuality. BR has long measured punctuality and monitored casualty rates (casualties being trains running late), and for the last few years it has set targets for each of its businesses and published its achievement against those targets. Again there is the problem of defining standards. The quality targets agreed with the Secretary of State in 1987 redefined a 'late' InterCity train as being ten minutes rather than five minutes late. And again, as the consultative committee points out, such figures are most useful when broken down into line-by-line figures (which BR does for its own internal consumption and, reluctantly, for the CTCC).

The internal purpose of measuring punctuality is twofold; for en route decision-making, such as whether to divert or delay trains, and for subsequent analysis. For the latter it is a long-established practice that the punctuality figures are circulated early the following day to the operations managers in the 'Daily Review of Operations' sheet. This PI has different uses according to time-scales: in the short term, management may make an immediate response, otherwise, these statistics are summarised four-weekly so that in the medium term they can be used for changing train plans and in the long term they inform the chief engineer's targets.

BR is currently updating the traditionally labour-intensive process of data collection by automating the system with the intention of releasing more high level staff to analyse the data. This will make it easier to compare actual and specified train times and to provide explanations for lateness, such as engine failure or bad weather. It will enable the analysis of specific routes such as Euston–Manchester and broad problems such as a high rate of engine failure across all lines and regions. Eventually it will be possible to debit the number of minutes lost and the cost of it on to specific lines, thereby enhancing strategic planning by informing the engineers of the value of faults so they can concentrate their resources on the most costly problems.

A further commercial use for punctuality PIs is to help BR compete in an increasingly competitive transport industry. For example, BR once monopolised the freight business but improvements in road transport mean that BR now has to battle just to retain core contracts for the transportation of mail and newspaper. Thus BR was compelled to build quality PIs into its contracts with the Post Office, promising repayment on a graduated scale if trains are late.

Considering this increasing interest in consumer issues, it is perhaps surprising that since 1986 BR no longer collates complaints on a national level; it is now the responsibility of each area manager to monitor complaints. This service is supplemented by the CTCC which monitors the complaints it receives and breaks them down into subjects. Thus the CTCC (1989) found that the most frequent complaint concerned the suitability of train services – 'reflecting unsatisfactory timetable changes and reductions in journey opportunities' (1989: 26) – information that is surely vital to a consumer-oriented organisation?

In contrast, there is a growing interest amongst BR management in obtaining customer perceptions and it has recently commissioned a number of surveys. These surveys consistently reveal the high regard that InterCity travellers attribute to punctuality and obtaining a seat whereas the commuter on Network SouthEast is most concerned about cancellations and punctuality. Some BR managers look abroad for ideas: in the Netherlands, for example, there is a sophisticated system containing around eighty quality PIs for passenger requirements. Quality objectives are specified and numerated, tasks are identified, and managers are accountable for their achievement; thus these quality objectives and PIs are explicitly incorporated into the management process. Crucially, however, the resources required to do it are underwritten by the Dutch Government. Without such a commitment, BR may only be able to develop such a system if it decides to redirect its strategy towards revenue-maximisation which would force it to pay greater attention to improving these effectiveness measures; until then, as one manager put it, 'quality performance indicators still tend to be tagged on by area managers as an afterthought to the main financial and productivity indicators'.

British Rail does seem to be several years ahead of other public sector organisations in the development of performance indicators. Where others are still awash with data-driven PIs, BR has learnt from its difficulties grappling with some two hundred PIs by drastically streamlining its system and incorporating them into explicit corporate objectives. In so doing, it has encountered serious problems in setting standards and disaggregating average figures – quite apart from the difficulty of actually achieving those targets. Despite this, British Rail provides an interesting example of an organisational learning process involving a move away from tin-openers *towards* dials. However, it also illustrates how the overriding priority of achieving governmental financial objectives has, in practice, resulted in an informal *hierarchy* of PIs in which external limits and rates of return are at the top and quality of service PIs are at the bottom. In short, as long as BR managers satisfy their financial targets, they can afford to undershoot their quality of service targets.

WATER INDUSTRY

The water industry is in a process of transition; as we completed our research the industry had just been privatised. All of our work was undertaken in the public water authorities formed when the previously disparate collection of some 1600 separate water undertakings were brought together in ten regional water authorities covering England and Wales in 1973; a 'monument . . . to technocratic rationality' (Day and Klein 1987: 135). The water authorities occupied a powerful monopolistic position. Not only is there a captive market because every consumer needs water but, despite the existence of twenty-eight statutory water companies supplying water to about 25 per cent of households (Vickers and Yarrow 1988), there was (and is) no supply-side competition within the industry.

The Water Act 1983 removed local authority representation on boards and made the industry fully nationalised, responsible to Parliament via the Secretary of State at the Department of the Environment (DoE) or, in the one case, for Wales. The regions retained some autonomy largely because of the dispersed nature of the industry, but the DoE exercised considerable central control, appointing all board members and treating the authority as 'an *essentially* managerial body, dealing with *essentially* technical rather than political problems, with members and officers as partners' (original emphases) (Day and Klein 1987: 137).

The water industry is concerned with the management of water. Two operational activities dominate the industry in terms of both costs and revenues: the supply of water to the consumer and the removal and safe disposal of waste, and these will be the focus of our analysis. But there are also a number of supporting functions such as environmental regulation – the control of river and drinking water, waste disposal, fisheries, and navigation – and the provision of community services including land drainage and flood protection. Despite this range of services the primacy of the supply of water and sewerage services makes it reasonable to describe the water industry as low on heterogeneity. Among all our organisations, the water industry is the most capital intensive but it still maintained a total workforce of some 50,000 in the ten authorities (Water Authorities Association 1986). It rates medium on complexity because there are a number of different skills: over half the workforce is graded as non-manual, a category that includes managerial, professional, technical, and craft skills. Although the existence of professional engineers and scientists alongside these other skills inevitably guarantees a degree of independence within the organisation, water rates no more than medium on autonomy. Significantly, as we shall see, water is clearly low on uncertainty. The relationship between inputs and outcomes is clear; if water does not run or sewers flood then there is no doubting the culprit. As we shall see, it is a service in which specific objectives can be set and achievement against those objectives can be monitored both quantitatively and qualitatively.

The design and use of performance indicators in the water industry

Given the structure of the industry and the nature of the service, we might expect the water industry to make considerable use of PIs. It is certainly the case that PIs have been around a long while: the 1945

Water Act provided that water should, subject to certain provisos, be constantly available in all supply pipes at a pressure sufficient to reach the highest point of the topmost storey of every building within the supply area; and, until 1979, the recommendations of the Royal Commission on Sewerage Disposal in 1912 still set standards for the discharge of sewerage and other effluents. But a number of political factors prompted an increase in the quantity, sophistication, and importance of PIs in recent years. Attention focused first on the financial performance of the water authorities. During the 1970s, it was a widely held assumption that the high capital intensivity of the water industry meant that operating costs were running at an optimum level. But times were changing and there were new constraints on public expenditure. Like British Rail, the water industry came under the ambit of the 1978 White Paper on Nationalised Industries. It responded immediately, symbolically, by publishing for the first time a set of national PIs in the 1978/9 Annual Reports of the ten regional authorities. This was followed by the imposition of external financial limits in 1978/9 and financial targets requiring a specific rate of return on assets in 1981/2. In 1981 the Department of Environment set out specific 'performance aims' which required individual water authorities to agree targets for operating costs during the three year periods finishing in 1983/4 and 1986/7. It is hardly surprising that the water authorities gave increasing importance to the development and improvement of financial PIs during this period.

The external pressure on financial and efficiency targets was matched, albeit to a lesser degree, by a growing concern about the quality of service. The Government insisted that the new performance aims should be achieved without any reduction in the level or quality of service, but how was this to be measured? The 1973 Water Act set out various objectives and functions that were translated into a number of performance targets: these included the need to secure 'an ample supply of water of appropriate quality to meet the growing demands of the people, industry, and agriculture – while at the same time ensuring that it is not wasted' and to achieve 'a massive clean-up of the country's rivers and estuaries by the early 1980s' (DoE 1973). These targets were rather vague and subjective – how were 'not wasted' and 'clean-up' to be defined and measured? A subsequent move towards more specific targets was encouraged by the growing significance of international quality standards, ranging from the World Health Organisation recommendations for 'European Standards for Drinking Water' to the stricter set of EC directives to which member states are now obliged to conform (WAA 1986: Ch. 5). Eventually the new imperative to report and account for performance led the water authorities to construct a set of 'level of service' PIs and since 1981/2 to publish planned level of service targets based on planned expenditure (WAA 1986: 24); this was a key step towards linking financial performance and standards of service.

When the Government introduced financial performance aims it originally intended to express them in terms of real costs per unit of output, but the industry objected that 'output could not be measured, and that even if it could be measured, its costs were related much more to the size of the system than to the throughput' (MMC 1981). In other words, there are several physical reasons why the costs of providing a service in one authority might differ from another. For example, where an authority has no access to the coast, such as Severn-Trent, the cost of the sewerage function is greater because it is much cheaper to discharge effluent into the sea. Rainfall varies between areas and over time so, to take an extreme example, a serious drought will have a profound, but differential, impact on the performance of individual authorities. Consequently, as the MMC continues: 'As a compromise, therefore, it was agreed that performance aims would be expressed in terms of total expenditure, with background information on movements in real unit costs measured by expenditure per head of effective population' (ibid.). The Government has, therefore, 'abandoned the attempt to assess the efficiency of any one water authority by comparing its costs to those of others. Instead, the emphasis is on looking at efficiency over time – as measured by the decline in unit costs – within each authority' (Day and Klein 1987: 141).

The Government did not escape criticism for this compromise: the Public Accounts Committee (1985) regarded the PIs as too imprecise to provide a satisfactory instrument for comparing the relative efficiency of water authorities. These financial PIs are mainly unit cost measures such as 'cost per head of equivalent population of operations' (and of manpower, chemicals, power, sewerage, etc.) involved in the supply and disposal of water, where 'equivalent' is the resident population plus an allowance for tourists and industry. However, these are average figures that do not seem to be disaggregated into PIs for specific tasks. Indeed, the MMC (1986) complained that, even in 1984, the Southern Water Authority was still unable to assess the unit costs of basic, day-to-day tasks such as repairing a burst main or reading a meter (although both the MMC and water industry managers reported that constant efforts were under way to improve these measures).

However, unlike many of the public sector services that we have studied, the water industry boasted an extensive set of performance indicators for measuring both the adequacy of the service to consumers and the quality of the product being delivered. There were twenty-five 'level of service' indicators which, although not fully comprehensive, covered all the basic functions of the water authorities – water supply, sewerage disposal, land drainage and flood protection, river quality, and recreational use (PAC 1985). The number of customers suffering from inadequate water pressure or from a supply failure of more than twelve hours was reported. Water quality was measured quantitatively by routine sampling of bacteriological and chemical concentrations, and qualitatively by monitoring sustained consumer complaints about 'colour, taste, smell or presence of "vehicle" animals (daphnae, shrimps, worms, etc.)'. The sewerage disposal PIs measured the number of premises flooded by foul sewerage, the number of sewer collapses, and the number of unsatisfactory storm overflows. Indeed, if anything the water industry is overflowing with effectiveness PIs.

These 'level of service' indicators had a variety of uses within the water industry. The DoE insisted that every water authority included them in the corporate plan which had to be approved by the DoE; consequently, all the planned objectives and targets were based on the level of service indicators. The DoE was able to draw on data from all the water authorities to assist it in deciding priorities. It could then use the PIs to try to ensure that performance aims were not being achieved at the expense of service quality. In particular, any significant gap between the plan and actual performance had to be explained by the water authority. Yet the DoE admitted to difficulties in monitoring closely the performance of individual authorities. There might be a 'seat of the pants feeling' that an authority was not performing which then prompted an examination of the PIs to provide evidence; particular attention being attributed to any failure to achieve the normative EC standards. But most of the figures had to be taken at 'face value' – the newness of the data meant that a satisfactory time-series was not yet complete. Moreover, the DoE only received aggregated information; it had no data on the distribution of performance within water authorities. So, for example, at the centre it was impossible to discover if all the breakdowns were in one area or were spread evenly throughout the region.

Consequently, the DoE tended to use PIs as tin-openers to 'trigger questions'. A particular concern was whether poor performance is 'an operational problem or an investment problem?' Put differently, is it a management fault or is it due to the poor state of the water authority assets – water works, sewers, etc. – in which case, the authority simply may not be capable of performing adequately. So the PIs can help assess the cost-effectiveness of alternative strategies. By asking how much of a plant fails to meet normative EC standards, it may be possible to isolate areas where it is worth spending on 'sensible replacement' or where capital investment is required.

But this raises a further complicating feature; even if it is a relatively straightforward task to determine that the solution to poor performance is capital replacement, it may still be a long time before performance can be improved. It can take twenty-five years to implement a programme for renewing a water mains system. At the operational level too there is often a time-lag between cause and effect. Even a burst mains takes time to affect service; indeed it may require the reporting of consumer complaints for staff to realise that there is a problem. On the other hand, the operational time-scale changes dramatically during a drought; a central control unit is established, detailed information is collected centrally on a daily basis, and swift actions, such as limiting the use of garden hoses, can have an immediate effect on performance.

PIs were also being used more frequently by individual water authorities. Initially, there was some discontent with the level of service indicators because, according to some water authority managers, 'We were measuring what we could measure; not necessarily what were the perceived areas of quality'. To overcome this problem, at least one authority developed a hierarchy of PIs, ranking them in order of importance; with only the aggregated indicators reported to the DoE. The 'key' PIs were the number and degree of interruptions to water supply, pressure, quality in terms of appearance, taste, and odour, and, for sewers, the number of foul floodings. These PIs were closely monitored and formed the basis of quarterly reports back to the executive of the water authority. Normative standards were set for these key PIs; for example, it was deemed unacceptable if a sewer flooded more than once in a two year period. One manager explained:

> Flooding only affects about 1300 properties a year but the experience is so unpleasant that we must make those homes falling into this 'unacceptable category' into priority cases. We isolate each case and set a financial target for preventative action on each property affected.

Similarly, when the water supply to the consumer breaks down, a good response time was defined as three hours, and an adequate response time was five hours. The intention was that those people falling into the lowest 'level four' category should become a priority for remedial action.

PIs were incorporated in Divisional Plans as formal targets and in many authorities they were examined monthly as part of the divisional monitoring package. Although there was uncertainty about how effectively managers were using this relatively new information, once a more reliable time-series is established, the credibility, and hence the use, of the level of service indicators should be enhanced.

Thus an important feature underlying the development and use of PIs by the water authorities (as opposed to the DoE) which contrasts with many of the other public sector organisations was that they had a strong prescriptive element; i.e. they assessed performance in terms of desired objectives, instead of merely comparing the activities of different authorities. This was possible because water authorities not only set specific objectives but could also monitor their achievement. Moreover, it is also possible quantitatively to measure quality of service; that is, the water authorities could measure performance against explicit standards of what the product should be like. Unlike, for example, the police or the NHS, there are normative standards involved in complying with EC statutory obligations for water quality and other services.

But even in the water industry there are no absolute standards; standard-setting is the result of a political process that has to weigh up what is both desirable and what is feasible, both technically and financially. In recent years, the water authorities have found it increasingly difficult to meet many of the exacting EC standards for water quality, river pollution, and designated safe bathing areas. The list of 'derogations' – applications for official permission not to meet a specific standard – is just one negative indicator of this failure. The cost of satisfying these standards was so great that in the run-up to privatisation Ministers were seeking to get some EC regulations relaxed. For example, the Government claimed that the EC directive on pesticide levels in water, which imposed a blanket ban limiting all pesticides in drinking water to under one part per million, had no proper scientific basis and was almost impossible to meet (*The Independent* 8 December 1988). Failure to meet this exacting standard produced the threat that the water authorities would be taken to court by the European Commission (*The Observer* 16 September 1989).

A further feature of the level of service indicators was that they were 'negative' PIs. Each PI recorded something that was undesirable about service delivery – chemicals or bacteria in water, burst mains, flooded sewers, effluent in bathing areas, and so on. As one manager complained, 'In an industry like gas or electricity it is possible to predict sales demand but in water this proves very difficult because it is the failures that create work for us rather than the demand for the service'. The emphasis on reacting to failures in the system meant that the water industry has always had a bottom-up orientation, largely because the widely distributed organisational structure has been associated with a highly devolved management system. The introduction of PIs allowed a shift towards a top-down structure because, as one senior manager observed, 'we have now developed the language that allows us to be more top-down; levels of service, performance indicators, they allow the service to lend itself more and more to performance review'. It is interesting that this same manager commented that 'the more distributed the workforce, the less control over quality'; he believed firmly that central control based on improved PIs allowed greater control over quality.

Turning to rivers, the responsibilities of the pre-privatisation water authorities were somewhat different. River quality was regulated by the authorities themselves, with lengths of river being classified on a six-grade classification (see Table 6.3). Apart from the water industry itself with its use of chemicals and discharging of waste, the main polluters of rivers are industry and farming; the uneven national distribution of industrial sites can be clearly detected in the longer stretches of Class 3 and 4 rivers in the North West and Yorkshire water authorities (WAA 1986). To a significant degree then, the authorities did not 'own' their performance in this area. This locational difference was probably exacerbated by the highly informal process through which water authorities tried to negotiate with individual firms in order to persuade them to refrain from discharging waste into rivers and to conform to environmental standards. Faced with the typical response

Table 6.3 Classification of rivers and canals

Class	
1A	waters of high quality suitable for potable supply abstractions and for all other abstractions; game or other high class fisheries; high amenity value.
1B	waters of less high quality than Class 1A but usable for substantially the same purposes.
2	waters suitable for potable supply after advanced treatment; supporting reasonably good coarse fisheries; moderate amenity value.
3	waters that are polluted to an extent that fish are absent or only sporadically present; may be used for low grade industrial abstraction purposes; considerable potential for further use if cleaned up.
4	waters which are grossly polluted and likely to cause nuisance.
X	insignificant water courses not usable where objective is to prevent nuisance developing.

Source: Water Authorities Association (1986) *Waterfacts*

from industry that either the pollution was not harmful, or that the proposed environmental controls would make the firm uncompetitive and hence threaten local jobs, it is clear that many managers opted for discretion and instigated a minimal number of legal actions against polluting firms and farmers (Environment Committee 1987). When an authority did take more cases to court, as did South West Water against farm pollution on the River Torridge in 1986, then they met powerful local resistance from the National Farmers Union (*The Independent* 16 October 1987).

Lastly, although level of service PIs were comparatively advanced in the water industry, managers still complained that useful, timely data are hard to obtain, particularly for individual properties. This encouraged some authorities to experiment in different ways of generating information. Some carried out a rather haphazard system of monitoring consumer complaints. Others commissioned consumer surveys to ascertain customer satisfaction and priorities. One authority instructed its workforce to take an 'optimal mark reader' on consumer visits which was used to build up a database of problems on individual properties because 'to link into the resource allocation system it is useful to locate exactly where problems exist and to obtain information on them'. This strategy generated some interesting information:

> previously we were dependent on simply monitoring aggregate numbers of customer complaints. Since implementing this new grass-root approach, we have been surprised by the level of dissatisfaction. For example, there was a significant difference between rural and urban complaints – urban dwellers are a lot more critical.

Although the water industry has long used PIs to measure basic levels of service, PIs became an increasingly important monitoring instrument during the 1980s. Like British Rail, the primary motivation was the government pressure to improve financial performance and productivity without impairing quality of service. Moreover, as PIs have become more reliable so managers have used them more frequently as a tool of managerial control at all levels of the organisation. A further boost for PIs will come from the introduction of performance-related pay. Currently, managers insist that 'performance indicators are used as a lever – they have no sanctions attached and there are no formal links with appraisal', but they recognise that following privatisation 'the next step is towards performance-related pay which may see a different use for PIs'. Severn-Trent was the first region to follow this path when it introduced bonuses 'aimed at promoting efficiency' (*The Guardian* 7 March 1989). In answering criticisms that cost-cutting bonuses could be detrimental to safety and quality standards, the chief executive of the authority declared that the scheme had been designed to ensure that new objectives for meeting more stringent quality targets would not be breached. It is as yet too early to pass judgement on this scheme.

However, the last point touches on another important development; the growing public concern about the quality of service. Two intertwined developments explain this changing environment: the escalation of interest in 'green' issues and the privatisation of the water industry. Growing awareness about environmental matters has prompted considerable concern about the performance of the water industry across a wide range of issues such as the level of nitrates and aluminium in drinking water, river pollution, and dirty beaches. Public anxiety was intensified by the debate accompanying the privatisation of the water industry. Indeed, so concerned was the Government to allay fears about the creation of a mammoth private monopoly that it set up a tough regulatory regime that, remarkably, was 'biased towards raising quality rather than controlling costs' (*The Economist* 24 March 1990). Thus the tightening of European Community rules on drinking water and sewage disposal will force the new water companies to pass on huge compliance costs to the consumer. There is a plethora of individuals and institutions responsible for regulating the industry ranging from the Secretary of State for the Environment, the Director-General of Water Services and Local Authorities, to the Drinking Water Inspectorate, the National Rivers Authority, and the Inspectorate of Pollution, all of whom will be monitoring some aspect of performance. Clearly, privatisation will serve only to increase the use and importance of performance indicators in the water industry.

BAA PLC

Prior to 1987 BAA was a nationalised industry conducting its business with its sponsor the Department of Transport, but in July of that year it was privatised. The main business of BAA is the operation of the three major south-eastern airports (Heathrow, Gatwick, and Stansted) and the four major Scottish airports. BAA handled 55.3 million passengers in the year to 31 March 1987 – about 73 per cent of UK air passenger traffic – and 85 per cent of UK air cargo tonnage (Vickers and Yarrow 1988). It is, in effect, a monopoly: major airlines have to use the London airports while BAA's commercial services have a captive market of travellers, often stranded by cancellations and delays, and always eager for duty-free bargains. By opting not to divide BAA into potentially competing parts, the Government engineered a privatisation that 'had virtually nothing to do with competition' (ibid.: 354).

BAA business falls into two areas. In 1987 some 48 per cent of revenue came from charges for airport traffic services provided to airlines; the rest was revenue from commercial activities. Most costs are incurred by traffic activities, so the secondary commercial activities provide a substantial cross-subsidy to the primary business of handling air traffic. The majority of the commercial activities are not handled directly by BAA but are franchised or sub-contracted to private sector firms – banks, retailers, newsagents, caterers, and so on; consequently, although BAA has around 7500 employees, this is only a tenth of the total number that work on BAA premises. Thus, despite the provision of a wide range of services – from parking aircraft to supporting Government functionaries such as customs and immigration – the franchising of commercial activity means that BAA is no more than medium on heterogeneity. Similarly, it is low on complexity because many of the skills on display on BAA premises are not those of BAA employees. BAA is also low on uncertainty because there is a clear relationship between inputs, outputs, and outcomes. There are clear lines of centralised authority within BAA, enhanced by the reorganisation of commercial activity into separate airport businesses. Airport managers are now responsible for all activities at an airport (MMC 1985). In one respect, there are serious problems regarding the ownership of performance, for many of the tasks carried out on BAA premises – immigration, customs, baggage (all of which are major sources of customer complaint) – are the responsibility of other organisations. Thus although there is little autonomy for individual units or workers *within* its own organisation, BAA finds itself in a sometimes awkward arm's-length relationship with its concessionaires, the airlines, and the various governmental departments that are located on its premises. Indeed, it is perhaps the most conspicuous example in our case studies of an organisation that does not own the performance of those services that matter most to its customers.

The design and use of performance indicators in BAA

The 1978 White Paper prompted BAA to clarify its objectives and to initiate a process of developing PIs. A set of draft objectives was agreed between the Government and BAA in 1983. The primary objective was 'to respond to the present and future needs of air transport in an efficient and profitable way by operating, planning, and developing its airports so that air travellers and cargo may pass through safely, swiftly, and as conveniently as possible'. Two further, linked policies played a significant role in the drive to develop PIs. First, the need to improve operating efficiency to meet government financial and performance aims, and BAA's external financing limits. Second, to improve the range and quality of services to customers and to follow the best practice of other airport authorities (a key yardstick given the monopoly position of BAA).

The quest for PIs was stimulated by two further factors. One was a report by the Monopolies and Mergers Commission (1985) into its commercial activities. BAA's monopolistic position creates a dilemma: if BAA maximises allocative efficiency by allowing competition between concessionaires supplying similar product ranges (e.g. rival bookshops) this would reduce BAA revenues by diminishing the value of the franchises. The Commission noted the potential danger of monopolistic abuse but, although expressing some concern about the attitude of BAA to competition, it did not feel BAA management was acting contrary to the public interest. Nevertheless amongst its recommendations the Commission suggested that BAA needed to 'develop more meaningful and specific indicators of performance' (4). Second, a number of BAA activities are closely regulated: safety and environmental regulation by the Civil Aviation Authority; airport charges come under various national (*Airports Act 1986*) and international agreements about non-discrimination between airlines of different nations; and there are five-yearly reviews by the Commission of 'operational activities'. Consequently, BAA needed robust PIs to enjoy an informed dialogue with these regulatory bodies.

BAA obviously makes use of conventional commercial PIs. In its evidence to the Monopolies and Mergers Commission, BAA argued that an increasing level of sales and profits provides an accurate medium and long-term reflection of customer satisfaction. The Commission accepted this point with the proviso that increases in revenue should be a result of passengers purchasing a higher number of goods and services and not simply due to higher prices. As noted above, the Commission also recommended that BAA should look at the performance of individual activities to ensure that levels of performance were consistent across all parts of the organisation.

The story of the process by which BAA came to improve its PIs is particularly relevant to the concerns of this book. It has been well described by Jim Brophy (1989), Financial Planning Manager at BAA, and in what follows we draw on his account. BAA began its search for

PIs by defining the business into four distinct areas each of which would require tailor-made PIs to monitor operating efficiency: the provision and utilisation of capacity; the generation of commercial income; the utilisation of manpower; and the standards of service provided to airport users.

The provision and utilisation of capacity reflects the basic function of BAA. Initially, four 'theoretical' PIs were selected as measures of this objective. Three of them – capital costs per unit of passenger capacity, utilisation of capacity provided, and the costs per unit of busy hour throughput – were unsatisfactory for evaluating overall performance. This was because it was necessary to aggregate the capacities of seven airports, all exhibiting different traffic patterns; for example, the long distance flights that dominate the load of Heathrow peak between 7am and 9am whereas the charter load of Gatwick is more evenly spread. While such PIs might be useful for building up a time-series to monitor change at individual airports, it would be difficult to use these aggregated figures to compare different airports. The fourth PI – passengers per unit gross asset – gave some indication of utilisation and allowed inter-airport comparison. However, the long lead-in times of investments in new facilities distort short-term figures; it was therefore discarded.

Instead, two proxy measures were adopted. First, the rate of return on net assets which, in a capital intensive industry, should show up any inefficient use of assets. Second, costs per passenger was chosen as a proxy for over-provision of facilities or under-utilisation of capacity by relating costs to the number of passengers handled. The PI is used to compare the performance of different locations and, by excluding depreciation and hence the distorting effect of differing asset values, comparisons can be made over time.

A similar process occurred in developing PIs for both the commercial and manpower areas: the problems of defining PIs and collecting data prompted a return to rather less ambitious proxy measures (see Table 6.4). Brophy argues that the lesson to be learnt from these exercises concerns the need to temper any ambition to construct perfect PIs and, instead, to focus on producing PIs that are relevant, comprehensible and useful to the manager.

BAA told the Commission that turnover provided 'an overall sense of a medium to long-term reflection of good service' (MMC 1985: 117) for its commercial activities. Digging deeper, it is clear that BAA managers found it very difficult to construct PIs for standards of service. Two areas were straightforward: safety posed little problem as there are minimum statutory requirements and speed of handling is assessed

Table 6.4 BAA financial performance indicators

Provision and utilisation of capacity:
Rate of return on net assets
Costs per passenger

Growth of commercial income:
Duty or tax free income per international passenger
Total income per terminal passenger
Growth in gross rental income

Utilisation of manpower:
Passengers per payroll hour
Costs per employee

Source: Brophy (1989)

according to the maximum time allowable for each process. But convenience is more complex and the measures more subjective.

It is complex because several key elements of performance are either outside the control of BAA, such as baggage delivery performance which is the responsibility of the airlines, or else performance is interdependent with other agencies, such as the time taken from aircraft arrival to passenger departure from the terminal which is influenced by the speed of baggage handling, passport controls, and customs. Various PIs are measured: for example, the MMC (1985) reported targets that 95 per cent of passengers should wait no more than three minutes at check-in, and that there was to be a period of no more than twenty-five minutes from the disembarkation of the first passenger to the collection of the last unit of baggage. But these targets are regarded internally as rather unsatisfactory indicators of performance because of the problems of performance ownership.

In 1983 out of ten broad BAA targets agreed between the Board and the Managing Director, there were just two relating to passenger service: the level of written complaints per 100,000 passengers and the 'availability of passenger sensitive mechanical equipment'. In other words, these were 'objective' PIs which could be measured; one target in 1984 was to have no more than fifteen complaints per 100,000 passengers. The main limitation of this PI arises from the inability of passengers to distinguish between those services provided by BAA, such as porters and information staff, and those provided by, for example, airlines, customs, and immigration authorities. It is also unlikely that dissatisfied customers, many of them foreigners, will be aware of the opportunity to complain. The second PI has proven more useful. It required the implementation of sophisticated technology to monitor passenger equipment such as passenger conveyors, lifts, and escalators for faults. The result was a highly effective negative PI providing an instant warning and diagnosis of problems that could also be fed into a target monitoring system; e.g. BAA can target (say) a 95 per cent reliability figure.

The problem with these 'objective' measures of what is actually provided is that it may not correspond with customer satisfaction. Therefore in 1983 BAA instigated at each airport a quarterly Passenger Opinion Survey based on a random selection of passengers. The survey aimed to discover the degree of use of a facility or service, the degree of satisfaction with it, and the extent to which views differ between categories of passenger. Brophy illustrates how this survey picked out catering and trolley services as areas within BAA's control that were generating considerable customer dissatisfaction. As a result various measures were taken to improve services – more trolleys and staff, catering outlets were diversified, and staff were trained in a 'Please the Passenger' campaign. Managers were given a target of 78 per cent departing passengers using landside catering to be 'satisfied'.

In 1983–4 two productivity indicators were used to set targets for managers: the costs per terminal passenger and the number of terminal passengers per payroll hour (MMC 1985). The intention was for PIs to be both a tool of management and a means of motivating managers; the targets were extended as far as middle management for the purposes of the Business Plan but down to lower levels for appraisal. By 1986 the BAA was able to use a number of PIs as an integral part of the new performance related pay system. The management bonus scheme pays a bonus based on profits, less a percentage for each performance target that a manager fails to achieve. Thus there are now five PIs for trolley availability, satisfaction, cleanliness, staff attitudes, and landside catering facilities, all of which are given targets that the responsible managers should pursue.

The BAA case also suggests that it is important to ensure that PIs are seen to be used at the highest level within an organisation. Before privatisation the PIs were used to agree targets with Government, to determine the payment of the Board Bonus and, later, the management bonuses. The PIs are now monitored on a monthly basis, with detailed six-monthly reports broken down by category (such as left luggage) and the key PIs, numbering between six and eight, are approved by the Board annually: 'if indicators are not used for management purposes, they will become theoretical rather than useful' (Brophy 1989: 2). Thus the decision to use PIs for performance related pay involved winning Board approval – 'selling it to top management' – and then 'cascading' the PIs and targets down the organisation. As Brophy observes, the evolution of this system took six years; it takes time to achieve anything and longer still to ensure the robustness of PIs that are to be built into a system of performance related pay. Nevertheless, as with British Rail, this is an interesting example of the development of a PI system over a number of years. In this case, BAA has not moved from a large number of PIs down to a small core; rather it has dispensed with meaningless or flawed measures and replaced them with a purpose-built set that has been carefully integrated into its management systems.

7 Performance indicators in the 1990s

Tools for managing political and administrative change

Perhaps the most helpful way to start reviewing the evidence of previous chapters is to return to the point of departure for our exploration. The Financial Management Initiative which prompted Whitehall's love affair with performance indicators hinged on the assumption that effective management in government required the definition of objectives and the development of measures to assess progress towards their achievement. So it would seem only reasonable, as a first step in moving towards our own conclusions, to ask whether the Government succeeded in achieving the policy objectives that prompted the whole exercise. What performance indicators can we devise to measure the success or otherwise of the Government's performance indicators crusade? The question is all the more illuminating because it turns out to be extremely difficult to answer. In making the attempt we illustrate, and summarise, some of the themes that have emerged during the course of the exploration: specifically, the complexities inherent both in the notion of defining objectives and in the design of performance indicators.

To start with, the Government's objectives in launching performance indicators turn out to be both multiple and ambiguous, with some evidence that they have shifted over time. The FMI exercise was itself, as noted in Chapter 1, a response to parliamentary criticism – drawing on a repertory of concepts and tools developed over the previous twenty years. The immediate objective might, therefore, be said to be to take symbolic action to meet criticism. If so, the indicator of success would be subsequent parliamentary approval, and the initiative would have to be judged a failure since it did not silence the Public Accounts Committee. But, of course, this is an inadequate account of the Government's objectives. It certainly would not explain the sustained dedication to the FMI programme in subsequent years. What we need, surely, is a more complex account of the Government's motives, distinguishing between the three, linked objectives outlined in the opening chapter. One important objective, clearly, was to achieve greater control over public expenditure and better value for money; another was to improve managerial competence in the public sector; a third was to bring about increased accountability as part of a movement towards greater decentralisation in the public sector.

If these were indeed the objectives, how would we devise indicators to tell us whether or not they have been achieved? How do we measure the progressive achievement of greater control over public expenditure or better value for money? On what scale do we assess the quality of public management? How do we quantify the degree of accountability? And, how, furthermore, do we identify the contribution of performance indicators or of any other component of the FMI programme in the achievement of these aims? To ask these questions is to identify a central dilemma in the use of performance indicators that has emerged from our exploration: indicators of policy *outcome* are hard to devise. And even when they are available, it is often impossible to disentangle the role of specific factors in bringing about a given outcome: so, for example, the control of public expenditure may reflect political decisions rather than the use of specific techniques. The 'ownership' of performance may be uncertain. Inevitably, therefore, it becomes necessary to fall back on indicators of *process* and *outputs*.

So, starting with process, we could measure the investment of effort by the Treasury and the Cabinet Office – for example, the number of special studies published – as well as the extent to which the production of performance indicators has become routinised in Whitehall. In these terms, government policy appears to have succeeded, although we might also note that the production of special studies seems to have fallen off in the last two years of the decade. Minimally, just as hypocrisy is the tribute by vice to virtue, so the production of performance indicators has become the tribute paid by Whitehall cynics to the Treasury. In this sense, then, performance indicators have become incorporated in the Whitehall culture. However, as with many process indicators, it is difficult to know whether they are measuring ritual or belief: the production of PIs may even be a substitute for performance.

Moving on to output indicators, the evidence of previous chapters would seem to suggest that government policy has been a run-away success. Year by year the number of departments and agencies producing PIs has increased; year by year, the number of such indicators has gone on rising. But, as we have also seen in previous chapters, such output or activity measures can be profoundly ambiguous. If doctors are performing more operations or if the police make more arrests, it does not necessarily follow that they are carrying out the most important operations or making the right arrests: output indicators may simply offer perverse incentives to carry out those activities where it is easiest to notch up a big score. And the same argument can be applied, of course, to the production of performance indicators themselves.

Patterns of implementation

If we are seeking understanding of the impact of the Government's initiative it may therefore be more illuminating to look at the way it has been implemented by the organisations studied rather than pursuing the elusive search for some indicators of overall success. What can we learn from the way in which PIs are devised and used in specific organisational settings, public and private? To what extent is their use contingent, as suggested in Chapter 2, on the particular characteristics of the organisations concerned? In what follows we seek to answer these questions: first by bringing together the evidence from the previous chapters and then by analysing the dynamics of the relationships revealed by the descriptive data.

Table 7.1 presents in summary form some of the main characteristics of the PI systems in the organisations studied. The first column shows whether the systems are based on data that pre-dated their invention (off-the-peg) or whether they developed their own database (bespoke). The second shows the speed of production: the range is from indicators that are available on a daily basis (contemporary) to those which only appear annually (historical). The third shows the quantity of PIs generated, on a scale from parsimony to promiscuity. We could, of course, have chosen or added other characteristics (for example, analysing PIs in terms of the conventional trinity of the three 'E's). But our strategy in this, as in other respects, has been to be ruthlessly selective in picking from the catalogue of categories and classifications laid out in Chapter 2. And our justification for concentrating on these three characteristics is that they help to discriminate among organisational attitudes towards the design of PI systems. So we would expect an organisation designing its PI system as part of a deliberate management strategy – as distinct from following the prevailing Whitehall fashion – to design its own data set, to want to have information quickly, and to concentrate on a handful of indicators linked to organisational objectives. Conversely, we would expect a conscript organisation to have a system driven by existing data, to be leisurely in its time requirements, and to hope that the sheer quantity of

Table 7.1 Characteristics of performance indicators in the case studies

Organisations	Design[1] Off-the-peg	/Bespoke	Timeliness[2] Slow	/Quick	Volume[1] Promiscuity	/Parsimony
Police	◆		◆		◆	
Courts	◆ →	◆		◆		◆
Prisons		◆	◆	◆		◆
Social Security		◆		◆		◆
NHS	◆		◆ ◆		◆	
Supermarket		◆		◆ ◆ ◆		◆
High Street Retailer		◆		◆		◆
Bank	◆ →	◆	◆			◆
Building Societies	◆ →	◆		◆		◆
Jupiter (TVhire)		◆		◆		◆
British Rail	◆ →	◆		◆	◆ →	◆
Water		◆		◆		◆
BAA	◆ →	◆		◆		◆

1 Arrows indicate the direction of change.
2 The more diamonds, the more emphatic the characteristic.

information would fudge the need for managerial decisions about aims and strategies.

Perhaps the single most significant conclusion to be drawn from Table 7.1 is that differences between organisations do not follow neatly the public/private divide. There are differences *within* each group: a point to which we return below. In terms of design, there is an almost even split between those organisations where the PI system is driven by the available data and those where the system dictated the data; a majority of private sector organisations, but not all, fall into the bespoke category while the public sector divides down the middle. In terms of timing, only two organisations – both in the public sector – fall into the historical category, i.e. relying on months-old data. And it is these same two organisations – the National Health Service and the police – which emerge in the 'promiscuous' column when it comes to the quantity of indicators used; British Rail, which was in the same category, has recently begun to move towards 'parsimony'. So it would seem that the second conclusion that can be drawn from the evidence is that the NHS and the police are somehow different from the other organisations studied.

Both conclusions are confirmed by Table 7.2. This shows the way in which PIs are used in different organisations by returning to one of the main distinctions made in Chapter 2. There it was argued that indicators can be used either as dials or as tin-openers. In the former case,

Table 7.2 Use of performance indicators in the case studies [1]

Organisations	Dials		Tin-openers
Police			♦
Courts		←	♦
Prisons			♦
Social Security		←	♦
NHS			♦
Supermarket	♦		
High Street Retailer	♦		
Bank		←	♦
Building Societies		←	♦
Jupiter (TVhire)	♦		
British Rail		←	♦
Water	♦		
BAA	♦		

1 Arrows indicate the direction of change.

'performance' can be read off the dials: that is, there is a set of norms or standards against which achievement can be assessed. These norms or standards may be either positive or negative; prescriptive or postscriptive. In the latter case, the indicators are simply descriptive. They do not speak for themselves. They may signal that a particular unit, be it district health authority, prison, or bank, is a statistical outlier, but no conclusions can be drawn from this fact in itself. It is simply an invitation to investigate, to probe, and to ask questions. Again, it is clear that differences do not follow the public/private distinction. Again, too, the table brings out the exceptionalism of the NHS and of the police. While our studies showed that nearly all the other organisations were beginning to move, if only tentatively, towards the prescriptive use of indicators – i.e. setting objectives or targets against which performance can be measured – the NHS and the police remain behind the pack. In this respect, however, they were joined by the prison service which, as Table 7.1 shows, has a bespoke, parsimonious, and quick PI system. All three continue to use PIs as tin-openers rather than as dials. In the case of the NHS, while targets are used in the annual review cycle between the Department of Health and the regional health authorities, these have not been incorporated in the PI package.

If the public/private dichotomy does not help us much in explaining the way in which organisations set about assessing their own performances, what does? The famous bottom line does not dictate convergence in the case of the private firms studied any more than its equivalent in the public sector, Prime Ministerial enthusiasm, brings about convergence among the departments and agencies examined. In the former case, the profit motive may be a key factor in explaining the commitment of private firms to devising a PI system, seen as a necessary condition for effective management. In the latter case, Prime Ministerial power may be the key factor in explaining the general trend towards the development of PI systems. So private profit and political power may be the respective – and very different – driving forces in the two sectors. But there is still differentiation within each sector. So, clearly, a more elaborate explanation is needed to account for the complex pattern revealed by the evidence. Accordingly, we return to our discussion in Chapter 2 of the various kinds of organisational characteristics which might plausibly be expected to be related to the design of PI systems. As in our previous analysis of the characteristics of the PI systems themselves, we do not attempt to go through the whole typological litany rehearsed in Chapter 2 but concentrate on those factors which seem most helpful in making sense of our findings.

Let us start with the two organisations, the NHS and the police, which stand out from the rest. In the former instance, just about all the factors liable to make the definition and measurement of performance problematic seem present. It is, to return to Table 2.1 (p. 34), high on heterogeneity, complexity, *and* uncertainty. That is, it is a multi-product organisation, which requires to mobilise a large cast with a high degree of interdependence between the different actors, and where the relationship between activity and impact is often uncertain. It is not always clear who 'owns' the performance; the activities of the NHS are only one of many factors influencing the health of the population. The overall objectives, even when defined, tend to be at a high level of generality. In addition, the principal actors involved – notably but not exclusively, the medical profession – enjoy a high degree of autonomy. The structure of authority is complex. The line of accountability from periphery to centre is clear in theory but, as we saw in Chapter 4, is often blurred in practice: indeed the introduction of PIs can be seen as part of a strategy to centralise knowledge about local performance while decentralising responsibility for the execution of government policies – centralising in order to decentralise, in Perrow's phrase (1977). All in all, despite some recent evidence of change (for example, PIs may soon be available on a monthly rather than yearly basis), the NHS thus stands out as the paradigmatic example of the organisational characteristics likely to produce a data-driven, slow, and promiscuous set of PIs, which are then used descriptively rather than prescriptively.

The police present many, though not all, of the organisational characteristics of our paradigmatic case. The service is low on complexity, medium on heterogeneity, and high on uncertainty. The ownership of performance is often uncertain; the principal actors, though lacking professional status, enjoy a high degree of autonomy; authority is divided between central and local government, and accountability is fuzzy. So the fact that the NHS and the police have a similar record when it comes to the design and use of PIs seems to vindicate our emphasis on organisational characteristics as important factors influencing the assessment of performance across and within the conventional public/private groupings. The point is further reinforced if we look at the other three 'service' agencies – Social Security, the courts, and the prison service – within the public sector. The profile of Social Security – low on heterogeneity, complexity, and uncertainty, with clear lines of accountability and a labour force that works within a set of very precise rules – resembles that of Supermarket which has perhaps the most sophisticated approach to PIs of all the organisations studied. Social Security has a bespoke system, relatively timely PIs, a parsimonious set, and is moving towards the development of targets or norms against which performance can be 'read off'. The prison service has, if anything, a more streamlined system but uses its PIs descriptively rather than prescriptively while, conversely, the courts have a less bespoke system but do have some dials. The latter two examples provide a mixed picture, of course, precisely because their organisational characteristics are less clear-cut than the other public sector agencies so far discussed: most notably, prison officers, like judges and barristers, probably enjoy almost as much autonomy as police officers and doctors.

All the public services so far considered are non-trading organisations. How important is this factor, as distinct from the 'public-ness' of the organisations concerned? To answer this question, we can turn to the public utilities. These are all services which sell their products or services. Like firms in the private sector they therefore have a 'bottom line': at the end of the year they have to account for their financial performance. And, as the two tables show, they are quite a homogeneous group: very much closer to the Social Security than the NHS model – with bespoke, relatively quick, and parsimonious PI systems, and sets of standards or norms against which performance can be 'read off'. But there are problems about interpreting this finding since it could be attributable to a variety of factors. Obviously, it could reflect the fact that they are in tradable sectors. But there may be other explanations as well. It could reflect the fact that the organisational characteristics of the utilities are much closer to Social Security than to the NHS; i.e. they tend to be low on heterogeneity, complexity, and uncertainty. It could reflect the fact that they have hierarchical authority structures and do not depend on professionals or others who have successfully asserted their autonomy. It could reflect the monopoly position of two out of the three utilities – water and BAA – which, as we saw in Chapter 6, creates the demand for a system of PIs designed to protect consumers against exploitation by giving visibility to the achievement of specific standards; and while the third, British Rail, is not quite a monopoly, it does have captive consumers on some commuter lines.

To disentangle these alternative – or possibly complementary – explanations, let us turn to the private sector firms. If the decisive factor were the 'bottom line', i.e. the fact these firms sell their goods or services, then we would again expect to find a homogeneous group. But, in practice, there are considerable variations within it. The contrast between Supermarket – the paradigmatic case at the opposite end of the scale to the NHS – and Bank is as great as that, say, between Social Security and the police in the public sector. Nor can this be explained in terms of organisational characteristics: in these terms Supermarket ought to be much closer to the NHS, while Bank should have a very similar profile to Social Security. If heterogeneity, complexity, and uncertainty were the decisive factors, indeed, the position of Supermarket and Bank should if anything be reversed. Two possible ways of resolving this puzzle are suggested by our evidence. The first revolves around the notion of performance ownership. In the case of Bank, as we saw, the branch manager's contribution to the performance of the organisation as a whole is severely limited: the level of profits is largely determined by the activities of head office; in contrast, in the case of Supermarket, the overall profits depend much more on the success of individual branches. The other factor identified by our evidence is the degree of competition. Supermarket operates in a highly competitive environment, with everyone in the organisation aware of the struggle for market shares. Bank was operating in what had, until recently, been a somewhat sleepy market, with customers inherited rather than won over. Indeed during the course of our study, the Bank was in the process of smartening up its PI system: a clear response to the increasingly competitive environment in which it found itself.

The case of Bank also underlines a more general point: the time dimension (Pollitt 1989). Most of the systems covered by our case studies were evolving and developing during the period of our enquiry, and no doubt have continued to do so since: we can predict with confidence that there will have been further changes even in the time between the completion of the field work and the publication of this book. Overall, the evidence suggests certain regularities in this pattern of organisational learning: a kind of innovations cycle. First, the pressures to introduce performance measurement lead to perfunctory compliance, expressed in the production (often over-production) of indicators – perhaps, as in the case of the NHS, through the mass baptism of existing statistics as PIs. Next, the production of PIs leads to resistance, notably attempts to discredit them by questioning their validity, timeliness, and appropriateness. There appears to be a standard repertory of denigration common to almost all the organisations studied. In response, refinements follow leading to the discovery that PIs may, after all, be useful – though not necessarily always in the ways intended by their designers (so, for example, the organisation may 'capture' the PI system in the sense that indicators are used to justify bottom-up claims for resources rather than as top-down instruments of control). Similarly, over time and with experience, indicators initially used as tin-openers may become dials. We do not wish to suggest that this cycle is inevitable in any deterministic sense or that all organisations will necessarily follow it, let alone that it is a normative or prescriptive model. Rather, we offer it as a warning of the possible traps involved in trying to explain the behaviour of changing organisations at one particular, necessarily arbitrary, point in time.

In summary, then, our evidence underlines the complexity of trying to understand the way in which different organisations set about assessing their own performance. No one explanation will do the trick. We can certainly dismiss the conventional view that the decisive factor is the presence or absence of a bottom line or the difference between organisations in the public and private sectors. We can, tentatively, suggest that internal organisational characteristics such as provider power and uncertainty about the relationship between means and ends tend to shape PI strategies in the public sector, while it is the degree of competition between organisations which is the chief driving force in the private sector. But our findings are a warning, if anything, about adopting any mono-causal explanation: the way in which PI systems will be shaped and used is contingent on a constantly changing environment, where new demands will create the need for adaptive organisational responses. The contingency is well-illustrated by one apparent paradox. This is that while monopoly will create pressure for more comprehensive PI systems in the case of public utilities, it will encourage private firms to take a rather sleepy approach. For in the first case there is a factor – political accountability and pressure – which does not exist in the second one: a factor which, as we argue in the concluding section of this chapter, may be expected to increase in importance in the 1990s.

Consumers and quality

Turning to dimensions of performance assessment not captured in our two tables, the evidence suggests that private sector firms and public utilities share one further characteristic which differentiates them fairly consistently from the public services studied. They are, for the most part, more consumer sensitive in the way they design their PI systems. First, these tend to include indicators aimed at measuring whether the *process* of providing goods or services is running smoothly and is tuned to consumer requirements. Are the shop shelves properly stocked? How often do the automatic cash pay-out points break down? How swiftly do the TV repairers call? Such indicators, as we have seen, may be either positive or negative. They may prescribe targets that should be achieved or they may sound alarm-bells when things occur that should not happen in a well-run organisation: for example, daphnae or shrimps in the water supply. Second, the PI systems often include indicators that seek to measure consumer satisfaction as an *output*, quite distinct from the sales figures: so, for example, complaints appear to be seen and used as a positive tool of management in a way which does not happen in the public sector. Similarly, consumer surveys are frequently used tools of performance appraisal: both Supermarket and High Street Retailer routinely use them to monitor consumer reactions to the way in which their branches are being run.

The finding would seem fairly predictable. Private sector firms, particularly in competitive markets, have good reasons to seek feed-back about their consumers: here again the famous 'bottom line' is a very inadequate indicator – if a very good incentive – since waiting for profits to dip as a signal of consumer discontent may be courting the risk of bankruptcy. Public utilities operating in competitive markets have much the same incentive. In contrast, monopoly public utilities – like the Water Authorities and BAA – do not. But here the explanation for the fact that they appear to be as consumer sensitive as private firms – at least in the design of their PI systems – is different. Consumer sensitivity (or at least the appearance of it) is the political price paid for their monopoly position. In effect, they are being required to demonstrate that they are not exploiting their captive consumers: in this respect, the way they assess their own performance has to be seen in the context of the wider regulatory systems within which they operate.

The public sector services studied also have their captive consumers, in some cases literally so. But the language of consumerism is somewhat at odds with the way in which these services have traditionally been perceived, not least by the providers. In effect, its use represents an attempt to subject and change the existing distribution of organisational power by carrying out a semantic revolution. So, for example, the linguistic transformation of the patient (someone to whom things are done: a passive concept) into a consumer of health care (someone who chooses and decides: an active concept), implicit in the Government's plans for the NHS, represents a major challenge to the service providers (Day and Klein 1989). In short, the language of the market place is being applied to organisations where none of the incentives of the market place exists. Their lack of enthusiasm is therefore entirely predictable and understandable. Additionally, public services face two problems which, if not unique to them, certainly appear to be especially intractable. The first is conceptual: multiple objectives reflect the existence of multiple consumer interest groups. The second is practical: how best to devise indicators of consumer reactions.

The first point is simply illustrated. Who are the consumers of police services? Is it those who have to call on their help, or those who look to them to maintain an environment in which their help is not required? Who, similarly, are the consumers of prisons? Is it those who are in gaol or those who see prisons as the bastions protecting society against crime? Who, lastly, are the consumers of the NHS? Is it those who actually use hospital and general practitioner services or those who see them as insurance against the day they have a heart attack? Indeed the instance of the NHS introduces a further twist into the argument. Satisfying customers who are interested in buying vegetables does not, in the case of Supermarket, mean frustrating customers who want to buy cheese. Nor does appealing to a new type of customer – someone who wants environmentally friendly products, perhaps – necessarily imply disappointing traditional shoppers. Even if, in the short run, space introduces an element of conflict, this can be resolved by building larger supermarkets – which is precisely the trend of recent years. In the case of public services operating with fixed budgets like the NHS, however, consumer groups are effectively in competition with each other for scarce resources: improving services for the acutely ill may be at the expense of services for the chronically ill. It is therefore possible to argue (Klein 1984) that a certain degree of insensitivity to consumer demands is positively desirable in order to protect the interests of those consumers with the least resources for either exit or voice – that is, the most vulnerable.

To make this last point is to identify a fundamental ambiguity in the concept of consumerism when applied to public services. In the private market place, consumerism is often taken to mean only the ability to signal demands for specific types of goods. If the consumers want more cars, and if they have the money to pay for them, they will get them. This, as suggested, creates problems when applied to the public sector, where resource decisions are made in the political market place. However, it is possible to apply the concept of consumerism in a different sense: that is, to apply it to process rather than outputs and the way in which services are delivered, rather than what is delivered. Here the difficulty is that of devising indicators of consumer reactions in public sector performance assessment: the practical question of how to devise instruments of measurement that are both affordable and timely. The difficulties can be illustrated by the example of the most ambitious attempt yet to elicit consumer reactions in the NHS (Prescott-Clarke *et al.* 1988). This population-based survey interviewed over 5000 people in four health districts. But given that only a small fraction of the population use the health services at any one point in time, the survey could not yield information about reactions to specific facilities: i.e. individual hospitals or surgeries. Nor, given the cost involved, could it be easily repeated, although we know that the delivery of health care is highly sensitive to such factors as staff turnover and morale, and that these may change very rapidly.

What this would suggest is that consumer surveys are mainly useful not as thermometers but as ways of generating standards which can then be incorporated in the routine collection of administrative data and the production of performance indicators. Long before the 1988 NHS survey, a series of studies had identified consumer concerns about the process of delivering health care (Cartwright 1983): excessively long waiting times for appointments and in out-patient departments, lack of information, the anonymity of medical staff, noise at night in wards, and so on. Indicators about many, if not all, such consumer concerns could have been incorporated in the NHS PI system long since, if there had been a willingness to collect the relevant information and, by so doing, to challenge the autonomy of the service deliverers. In fact, such indicators are now about to come in by the back-door, not as part of the NHS PI system but as part of the move towards making contractual arrangements for the delivery of all services. These will incorporate requirements about the standards of the services that are to be delivered as part of the contract: these may specify, for example, the average waiting time for appointments or in out-patient departments that is to be achieved (Department of Health 1990). So, as part of the new contract system, the NHS may move towards having a set of targets or norms, against which performance can be 'read off'.

But will the way in which performance is defined include a *quality* dimension? As we saw in Chapter 2, one of the criticisms made of PIs in the public sector is precisely that they tend not to measure quality. But, before trying to answer this question, it is worth analysing the concept of 'quality' itself in the light of what we have learnt from previous chapters. There are indeed quality indicators to be found in the PI systems that we have reviewed. So, in the case of water, it is possible to define and to test directly various aspects of quality: purity and taste, for example. In the case of Supermarket and High Street Store, too, it is possible to test the goods to ensure that they have achieved specified quality standards. The difficulties begin where service *is* the product or one of the elements in it. In these cases, it is not self-evident that 'quality' is something identifiable in its own right as distinct from being the by-product of other activities that are being carried out. Quality, in this sense, can perhaps best be seen as the result of competence in the routine activities of the organisation: something, in short, which permeates all activity and is integral to everything that happens, as distinct from being an add-on-extra. It may still be possible to have negative or prescriptive indicators which signal that competence has not been achieved. If there is an excess of mortality or morbidity following NHS operations, in a given hospital this may well be a signal that the quality of medical care is deficient. But, more often, the real indicators of quality will be that the ordinary, routine things are being done properly and on time. So, for example, the indicator measuring the proportion of emergency ambulance calls which meet response time standards (Table 4.7, p. 110) can be seen as a quality indicator in this larger sense. Again, in the case of the NHS the move towards contracts will create new opportunities for introducing indicators of this type (Hopkins and Maxwell 1990). Nor are such process indicators necessarily to be dismissed as second best, to be tolerated only in the absence of the outcome measures which will eventually make them redundant. Developing outcome measures is, at best, very difficult and may, in some cases, turn out to be a search for the chimera. Moreover, in some circumstances process indicators may actually be more relevant and more significant: the outcome of long stay geriatric care is almost always death – and what really matters is the quality of the process leading up to it.

In concentrating on the case of the NHS to illustrate the problems of introducing a consumer perspective and quality indicators we have deliberately concentrated on conspicuous 'laggards' in these respects among the organisations studied. In doing so, we have also come back once more to one of our recurring themes: the importance of organisational factors in determining the way in which PI systems are designed and function. In the instance of the NHS, it is largely the degree of professional autonomy enjoyed by the service providers which has hitherto constrained the adoption of PIs that might be perceived as a threat to (because, in part, a measure of) the prevailing way in which the service providers carry out their functions. In contrast, Social Security has managed to use consumer surveys to help generate both targets of performance and ways of assessing quality, defined very much in our sense of doing routine things well and promptly. Given the very different status and power of the service providers, this is a predictable outcome and entirely consistent with our emphasis throughout on the differentiating impact of organisational factors within the public sector. However, to stress only organisational characteristics would be an overly deterministic conclusion to our study. These characteristics are not cast in concrete for all time. PI systems in the public sector are largely organisational responses to outside stimuli, as we saw in Chapter 1. They were mostly prompted by signals from the political environment in the first place. And political pressure or turbulence has, in fact, been a continuing stimulus to change and innovation since the original FMI push. So, in the case of Social Security, the stimulus came partly from criticisms by the National Audit Office and partly from an impending move towards decentralisation and agency status. In the case of prisons, a spur came from political apprehension about the consequences of television making a regular feature of prisoners showering tiles on their gaolers. Similarly, in the case of the NHS new possibilities have opened up as a result of larger changes: specifically, from the move towards a contract culture and the implicit challenge to the traditional position of the service providers. In the final section of this chapter, we therefore turn to examining the larger forces that may shape the development of performance assessment in the public sector during the rest of the 1990s.

Prospects for the 1990s

Looking back over the recent history of innovation in British government, the first chapter suggested that the introduction of such new initiatives as the FMI and such new techniques as PIs represented a resurrection rather than a revolution. The evidence reviewed there suggested that attempts to reform the management of government follow a cyclical pattern: enthusiasm followed by disillusion and oblivion which, in due course, leads to re-discovery. This prompts some uneasy questions. In reviewing the developments of the 1980s in the previous chapters, have we been reporting on a flourishing industry or writing an obituary on an experiment that is about to go the way of its predecessors? Will the FMI and PIs join, in the 1990s, long forgotten acronyms like PPB and PAR? How dependent has been the wave of enthusiasm for performance assessment in Whitehall on the personality of a particular Prime Minister, or a particular style of party government, and will it wane as these change? For what purposes will PIs be used in the 1990s, by whom, and with what audience in mind? What, in Richard Rose's phrase (1972), will be the market for indicators?

The best way of starting to answer these questions is, perhaps, to examine 'the most ambitious attempt at Civil Service reform in the twentieth century' (Treasury and Civil Service Committee 1990: v). This is the Next Steps Initiative, which has taken over from the Financial Management Initiative as the banner of reform in Whitehall. Its origins and its name derive from a report of the Prime Minister's Efficiency Unit (Jenkins *et al.* 1988). This shifted the emphasis from change *within* the existing structure of government to change *of* the structure itself. The theme of policy at the start of the 1990s was how best to transfer responsibility for service delivery from Whitehall to agencies, with Ministers and their civil service advisers concentrating on 'their proper strategic role of setting the framework and looking ahead to plan policy development' (17). Enthusiastically backed by Mrs Thatcher (and later endorsed by Mr Major), Next Steps prompted an ambitious programme of decentralisation. By mid-1990, thirty-three agencies had been established: many more were in the pipeline. So, for example, the Department of Social Security – the biggest Whitehall Ministry, in spending terms – was about to be split into a series of service delivery agencies. By the summer of 1991, there were some fifty agencies with a total staff of 200,000, i.e. about half of the Civil Service (Treasury and Civil Service Committee 1990: vi). It seems a development likely to survive swings in both fashion and political control. Not only do its intellectual roots go back to the Fulton Committee, but it has widespread support cutting across political parties, including that of the bi-partisan Treasury and Civil Service Committee whose report has already been quoted.

All this would suggest that the displacement of FMI by Next Steps will, if anything, increase the role of performance indicators and reinforce interest in developing them further in the 1990s. If central government is to maintain control over the implementation of policies while at the same time decentralising day to day responsibility, then PIs become an essential tool: it is necessary to centralise knowledge about key aspects of performance in order to be able to decentralise activity. The point is easily illustrated. The key step in setting up an agency is to draw up a Framework Agreement which sets out its status, aims, and objectives. From this then flows a set of performance targets. So, for example, the Driving Standards Agency is required to reduce waiting times for driving tests to a national average of eight weeks and to achieve an examiner utilisation rate of 72 per cent, among other targets. In short, the notion of PIs – designed to assess performance both in terms of the standards of service to be achieved and the efficient use of resources – is integral to the whole process of setting up agencies under the Next Steps Initiative.

There are other reasons, too, for expecting PIs to become increasingly important as tools of public (as well as private) management and control. To a large extent, as already argued, they are the children of information technology: one of the key differences between the 1960s (when PIs were first conceived, as shown in Chapter 1) and the 1980s (when they finally flourished) was precisely that the price of the new technology had dropped while its virtuosity and diffusion have accelerated in the intervening years. As the diffusion of the technology continues in the 1990s – and, perhaps more important, its use becomes routinised – so it seems reasonable to predict greater use of PIs at all organisational levels. But, of course, the role of technology is only an enabling one: the opportunities it offers for innovation in the way we think about political, administrative, and managerial issues. More important in the 1990s may, therefore, be the growing political interest in regulation as an instrument of government. The paradox of privatisation in the 1980s, as already noted, is that it led to an increase in government regulation: there was a growth of new regulatory agencies responsible for policing the newly privatised water, telephone, and other concerns. And PIs are an essential instrument of regulation. Similarly, the changes in the NHS following the 1989 Review (Day and Klein 1989) will turn district health authorities into pur-chasers of health care, contracting to buy services from hospitals. Such contracts – like Framework Agreements – will have to specify the performance required, and indicators will have to be devised to assess whether or not quality standards or output targets are being achieved. And there are parallel changes in the personal social services.

To stress the scope for the development of PI systems in the 1990s is also to underline the importance of debate about how they should be designed and used. PI systems are likely to grow in importance precisely because they are a response to a variety of policy concerns: they are instruments which can be designed and used to serve different objectives. In the past, to return to the distinction made at the beginning of this chapter, the development of PIs was driven by three sets of linked preoccupations: the control of public expenditure, managerial competence, and greater accountability. To this has now been added interest in decentralisation or 'hands-off' control by government

(Carter 1989). PI systems cannot therefore be seen as neutral technical exercises: toys for the experts, as it were. Given different policy objectives, different kinds of PI systems will emerge. So, for example, if the prime concern is with the efficient use of public resources, the emphasis will be on trying to devise output (and, if possible, outcome) measures: the approach of the economist, as we saw in Chapter 2. If the prime concern is with accountability, then a rather different emphasis may emerge: process indicators which measure the way in which services are delivered to the public – their availability, their timeliness, and their appropriateness – may be more relevant. If the focus of attention is on managerial competence, then the stress may be on setting targets for the performance of individual units or branches.

These objectives may, of course, co-exist within the same organisation. Different organisational actors, operating at different levels of the organisation, may vary in the relative emphasis they put on them. As we have seen, PIs can be used for different purposes even within the same organisation: in some cases, notably the NHS, they are little more than a data bank into which various actors dip as and when it suits their purposes. Moreover, there is clearly a tension between PIs seen as instruments of hierarchical, managerial control – accountability to the top – and PIs seen as aids to self-monitoring and self-examination by those involved in service delivery. Here, once again, the role of technology is central. To the extent that a PI system like Supermarket's can give almost instant visibility to the activities of those involved at the organisational coalface, so it threatens to limit their discretion and autonomy. In short, it may imply a change in the balance of power between organisational actors (Zuboff 1988). As and when the public sector moves in the same direction – and there is no technical reason why the Secretary of State for Health should not soon be able to have a list of operations carried out in each health district on his desk the day after they were performed – so, clearly, there will be potential for a much more direct dialogue between centre and periphery.

It is a dialogue which could, all too easily, turn into a confused babble of voices. Not only are PIs the children of information technology, but they can also be its victims in the sense that the capacity for handling and transferring vast quantities of data quickly may outstrip the capacity of the organisational system, and of the individuals within it, to handle them. To an extent, this has happened already in the public sector. As noted already, the public sector – in contrast to the private sector – tends to be conspicuous for the promiscuous proliferation of its PIs. In so far as this reflects the complexity and heterogeneity of the organisations concerned – and the uncertainty about the relationship between inputs and outputs (not to speak of outcomes) – this may be inescapable. But to the extent that it simply reflects an organisational response to the demand for the production of PIs – that it represents taking the easy way by re-labelling existing data as PIs – so it becomes a source of confusion. All too easily such a response can become a substitute for defining objectives and measuring achievements. So, for instance, it would be disastrous if the Secretary of State for Health were to get information about every operation performed: the need is for an indicator which tells him or her about the extent to which policy objectives – for example, the reduction of waiting times – are being achieved. In this respect, the lesson to be drawn from the experience of the private sector is unambiguous and clearly applicable to the public sector: there is virtue in parsimony as an aid to understanding and as a necessary condition for making a PI system usable.

To emphasise the crucial importance of making PI systems usable – to argue for designing such systems with the needs of their consumers in mind – is to do more than to underline yet again the desirability of parsimony, timeliness, and comprehensibility. It is also to ask the question, who are, or should be, the consumers of PIs? Where will the demands for their production and consumption come from? Our analysis has already suggested some of the answers. Demands will come from Ministers and Whitehall civil servants as they strive to maintain control over activities that are being hived off; demand will come, too, from middle managers who see PIs as a mirror in which to examine their own performance. Finally, demand may come if PIs are seen as instruments of accountability not only *within* organisations – their present purpose, and the reason why they were invented in the first place – but as ways of making organisations accountable for their collective performance. Here the model may well be provided by the public utilities which have moved into private ownership: the result, as we have seen, has been a demand for indicators of performance to complement the bottom line and to ensure that profits are not being achieved by exploiting consumers in a monopoly situation.

Surprisingly, however, Parliament has yet to emerge as an effective consumer. In this respect, the 1980s mark a surprising failure. As a result of the FMI, the Government's annual Public Expenditure White Paper (Carter 1988) is, as already noted, punctuated by PIs. Indeed the number for PIs has achieved epidemic proportions. But although the White Paper is supposedly the Government's explanation of its financial stewardship to Parliament, there has been surprisingly little interest among MPs in performance indicators. Despite the occasional paragraph in the reports of Parliamentary Committees, MPs generally have demonstrated massive indifference and boredom. Performance indicators have been seen as technical instruments at best and propaganda at worst, and in any case incomprehensible or misleading. There has been no real attempt to use them as instruments of parliamentary accountability: to ask the question of how the performance of government should be measured and what indicators are needed. Yet this, surely, is what parliamentary accountability is all about – in theory, at least.

Here, then, is the agenda for the 1990s: to rescue the concept of PIs from the experts and to see whether, and how, it can be integrated into the democratic process. In making the attempt, the design of PI systems will have to change to make them accessible to new audiences; the concept itself may well evolve and widen; possibly even, new words may have to be found for it. Certainly extra dimensions of performance may come to be included: for example, distributive equity in service delivery to complement efficiency. But if, by the end of the 1990s, PIs as such have become part of the linguistic history of reform in British government but the notion of seeking ways of explicitly assessing the performance of government has taken hold, then no one will mourn. The real challenge is to move from an exclusively managerial view of accountability and the role of performance indicators, to a wider, political definition.

References

Abel-Smith, B. (1973) *Accounting for Health*, London: King Edward's Hospital Fund.

Aldrich, H. (1972) 'Technology and organizational structure: a re-examination of the findings of the Aston Group', *Administrative Science Quarterly* 17: 26–42.

Audit Commission (1986) *Performance Review in Local Government*, London: HMSO.

Banks, G.T. (1979) 'Programme budgeting in the DHSS', in T.A. Booth (ed.) *Planning for Welfare*, Oxford: Basil Blackwell.

Barratt, R. (1986) 'The way ahead: inspectorate or directorate?', address to the conference of the *Association of Chief Police Officers*, 11 June.

Beard, W. (1988) 'Information technology in the public service', in P. Jackson and F. Terry (eds) *Public Domain 1988*, London: Royal Institute of Public Administration.

Bexley, London Borough of (1985) *Annual Review of Service Performance 1984/85*.

Birch, R. (1989) 'Target setting and performance measurement in Social Security', text of a speech prepared for the *Strategic Planning Society*, May.

British Railways Board (1981) *Productivity Report*, mimeo.

British Railways Board (1982) *Productivity Performance*, London.

British Railways Board (1987) *Corporate Plan*, London.

British Railways Board (1988) *Annual Report and Accounts 1987/88*, London.

British Railways Board (1989) *Annual Report and Accounts 1988/89*, London.

Brophy, J. (1989) 'Performance indicators in the public sector: a case study – BAA plc', paper presented at the *Strategic Planning Society*, May.

Buswell, D. (1986) 'The development of a quality-measurement system for a UK bank', in B. Moore (ed.) *Are They Being Served?*, Oxford: Philip Allan.

Butler, T. (1985) 'Objectives and accountability in policing', *Policing* 1, 3: 174–86.

Butt, H. and Palmer, B. (1985) *Value for Money in the Public Sector: the Decision Maker's Guide*, Oxford: Basil Blackwell.

Carter, N. (1988) 'Measuring government performance', *Political Quarterly* 59, 3: 369–75.

Carter, N. (1989) 'Performance indicators: "backseat driving" or "hands off" control?', *Policy and Politics*, 17, 2: 131–8.

Cartwright, A. (1983) *Health Surveys*, London: King Edward's Hospital Fund.

Cave, M., Hanney, S., Kogan, M., and Trevitt, G. (1988) *The Use of Performance Indicators in Higher Education*, London: Jessica Kingsley.

Central Transport Consultative Committee (1988) *Annual Report 1987–88*, London.

Central Transport Consultative Committee (1989) *Annual Report 1988–89*, London.

Chadwick, E. (1867) 'On the chief methods of preparing for legislation', *Fraser's Magazine* 27 May: 673–90.

Challis, L., Fuller, S., Henwood, M., Klein, R., Plowden W., Webb, A., Whittingham, P., and Wistow, G. (1988) *Joint Approaches to Social Policy*, Cambridge: Cambridge University Press.

Chancellor of the Exchequer (1961) *Control of Public Expenditure*, London: HMSO, Cmnd. 1432.

Chaplin, B. (1982) 'Accountable regimes: what next?', *Prison Service Journal* October: 3–5.

Chief Inspector of Constabulary (1989) *Report, 1988*, London: HMSO, HC 449.

Christian, J. (1982) *A Planning Programming Budgeting System in the Police Service in England and Wales between 1969 and 1974*, unpublished M.A. thesis, University of Manchester.

CIPFA (1984) *Performance Indicators in the Education Service*, London.

Clarke, P. (1984) 'Performance evaluation of public sector programmes', *Administration*, 32, 3: 294–311.

Clarke, R. and Cornish, D. (eds) (1983) *Crime Control in Britain*, Albany: State University of New York Press.

Clegg, S. and Dunkerley, D. (1980) *Organization, Class and Control*, London: Routledge & Kegan Paul.

Collins, K. (1985) 'Some issues in police effectiveness and efficiency', *Policing* 1, 2: 70–6.

Conservative Central Office (1979) *The Conservative Manifesto*, London: Conservative Central Office.

Crick, B. (1968) *The Reform of Parliament*, 2nd edition, London: Weidenfeld & Nicolson.

Cyert, J. and March, J. (1963) *A Behavioural Theory of the Firm*, Englewood Cliffs, NJ: Prentice-Hall.

Day, P. and Klein, R. (1985) 'Central accountability and local decision making', *British Medical Journal* 290, 1 June: 1676–8.

Day, P. and Klein, R. (1987) *Accountabilities*, London: Tavistock.

Day, P. and Klein, R. (1989) 'The politics of modernisation: Britain's National Health Service in the 1980s', *Milbank Quarterly* 67, 1: 1–35.

Department of Education and Science (1970) *Output Budgeting for the DES: Report of a Feasibility Study*, London: HMSO.

Department of Environment (1981) *Local Authority Annual Reports*, London: HMSO.

Department of Environment and Welsh Office (1973) *A Background to Water Reorganization in England and Wales*, London: HMSO.

Department of Health (1990) *Contracts for Health Services*, London: HMSO.

Department of Health and Social Security (1972) *Report on Confidential Enquiries into Maternal Deaths in England and Wales 1967–1969*, London: HMSO.

Department of Health and Social Security (1981) *Care in Action*, London: HMSO.

Department of Health and Social Security (1986) *Performance Indicators for the NHS: Guidance for Users*, London: DHSS.

Department of Health and Social Security (1988) *Comparing Health Authorities*, London: DHSS.

Dunbar, I. (1985) *A Sense of Direction*, London: Home Office.

Dunleavy, P. (1989) 'The architecture of the British central state', *Public Administration*, 67, 3: 249–75.

Dunsire, A., Hartley, K., Parker, D., and Dimitriou, B. (1988) 'Organizational status and performance: a conceptual framework for testing public choice theories', *Public Administration* 66, 4: 363–88.

Electricity Council (1988) *Performance Indicators 1987/88*, London.

Environment Committee (1987) *Pollution of Rivers and Estuaries* (3rd Report, Session 1986–87), London: HMSO HC 183–1.

Evans, R. (1987) 'Management, performance and information', *Prison Service Journal* April: 9–12.

Expenditure Committee (1971) *Command Papers on Public Expenditure*, Third Report, Session 1970–71, London: HMSO, HC 549.

Expenditure Committee (1972) *The Relationship of Expenditure to Needs*, Eighth Report, Session 1971–72, London: HMSO, HC 515.

Ferner, A. (1988) *Governments, Managers, and Industrial Relations*, Oxford: Basil Blackwell.

Flynn, A., Gray, A., Jenkins, W., and Rutherford, B. (1988) 'Making indicators perform', *Public Money and Management* (winter): 35–41.

Flynn, N. (1986) 'Performance measurement in public sector services', *Policy and Politics* 14, 3: 389–404.

Fulton, Lord (1968) *The Civil Service: Report of the Committee*, London: HMSO, Cmnd. 3638.

Garrett, J. (1980) *Managing the Civil Service*, London: Heinemann.

Goldman, H. (1984) 'Prisons and performance measurement', *Research Bulletin (Home Office Research and Planning Unit) No.18: 36–8.*

Gray, J. and Jesson, D. (1987) 'Exam results and local authority league tables', in A. Harrison and J. Gretton (eds) *Education and Training UK 1987*, Newbury: Policy Journals.

Guillebaud, C. (1956) *Report of the Committee of Enquiry into the Cost of the National Health Service*, London: HMSO, Cmnd. 9663.

Harrison, A. and Gretton, J. (1986) 'The crime business: a growth industry?', in A. Harrison and J. Gretton (eds) *Crime UK 1986*, Newbury: Policy Journals.

Health Services Indicators Group (1988) *A Report on Körner Indicators*, London: DHSS.

Heclo, H. and Wildavsky, A. (1981) *The Private Government of Public Money*, 2nd edition, London: Macmillan.

HM Chief Inspector of Prisons (1982) *Annual Report 1981*, London: HMSO.

HM Treasury (1978) *The Nationalised Industries*, London: HMSO, Cmnd. 7131.

HM Treasury (1986a) *Output and Performance Measurement in Central Government: Progress in Departments* (ed.: S. Lewis), Treasury Working Paper No. 38, London, February.

HM Treasury (1986b) *Multidepartmental Review of Budgeting: Final Central Report*, (ed.: A. Wilson *et al.*), London, March.

HM Treasury (1987) *Output and Performance Measurement in Central Government: Some Practical Achievements* (ed.: P. Durham), Treasury Working Paper No. 45, London, January.

HM Treasury (1988) *The Government's Expenditure Plans 1988–89 to 1990–1991*, 2 Volumes, London: HMSO, Cmnd. 288.

HM Treasury (1990) *The Government's Expenditure Plans 1990–91 to 1992–1993*, London: HMSO, Cmnds 1001, 1008, 1009, 1013, 1014.

Heseltine, M. (1987) *Where There's a Will*, London: Hutchinson.

Hill, M. and Bramley, G. (1986) *Analysing Social Policy*, Oxford: Basil Blackwell.

Hitch, C.J. (1965) *Decision-making for Defense*, California: University of California Press.

Home Office (1979) *Committee of Inquiry into the UK Prison Services* (The 'May Report'), London: HMSO, Cmnd. 7673.

Home Office (1983) *Manpower, Effectiveness and Efficiency in the Police Service*, Circular 114/1983, London.

Home Office (1984) *Management in the Prison Service*, Circular 55/1984, London.

Hood, C. and Dunsire, A. (1981) *Bureaumetrics*, Aldershot: Gower.

Hopkins, A. and Maxwell, R. (1990) 'Contracts and quality of care', *British Medical Journal* 300, 7 April: 919–22.

Hopwood, A. (1984) 'Accounting and the pursuit of efficiency', in A. Hopwood and C. Tomkins, *Issues in Public Sector Accounting*, Oxford: Philip Allan.

Jackson, P. (1988) 'The management of performance in the public sector', *Public Money and Management* (winter): 11–16.

Jackson, P. and Palmer, A. (1988) 'Extending the frontiers of performance measurement: how much further can we go?', in D. Beeton (ed.) *Performance Measurement: Getting the Concepts Right*, Discussion Paper 18, London: Public Finance Foundation.

Jenkins, K., Caines, K., and Jackson, A. (1988) *Improving Management in Government: The Next Steps*, London: HMSO.

Jenkins, L., Bardsley, M., Coles, J., Wickings I., and Leow H. (1987) *Use and Validity of NHS Performance Indicators: A National Survey*, London: CASPE, King Edward's Hospital Fund.

Joint Consultative Committee (1990) *Operational Policing Review*, Surbiton: JCC.

Jones, S. and Silverman, E. (1984) 'What price efficiency? Circular arguments. Financial constraints on the police in Britain', *Policing* 1, 1: 31–48.

Jowett, P. and Rothwell, M. (1988) *Performance Indicators in the Public Sector*, London: Macmillan.

Kanter, R. and Summers, D. (1987) 'Doing well while doing good: dilemmas of performance measurement in nonprofit organizations and the need for a multiple constituency approach', in W. Powell (ed.) *Handbook of Nonprofit Organizations*, New Haven, CT: Yale University Press.

King, A. (1975) 'Overload: problems of governing in the 1970s', *Political Studies*, 23, 2–3: 284–96.

King, R. and Morgan, R. (1980) *The Future of the Prison System*, London: Gower.

Klein, R. (1972) 'The Politics of PPB', *Political Quarterly*, 43, 3: 270–81.

Klein, R. (1982) 'Performance, evaluation, and the NHS: a case study in conceptual perplexity and organizational complexity', *Public Administration* 60, 4: 385–407.

Klein, R. (1984) 'The politics of participation', in R. Maxwell and N. Weaver (eds) *Public Participation in Health*, London: King Edward's Hospital Fund.

Klein, R. (1985) 'Health policy, 1979–1983', in P. Jackson (ed.) *Implementing Government Policy Initiatives: The Thatcher Administration 1979–1983*, London: Royal Institute of Public Administration.

Klein, R. (1989a) 'Money, information and politics', in David Collard (ed.) *Fiscal Policy: Essays in Honour of Cedric Sandford*, Aldershot: Gower.

Klein, R. (1989b) *The Politics of the NHS*, 2nd edition, London: Longman.

Levitt, M. and Joyce, M. (1987) *The Growth and Efficiency of Public Spending*, Cambridge: Cambridge University Press.

Lloyds Bank Economic Bulletin (1988) No. 119, November.

Lord, R. (1987) 'Re-writing the Public Expenditure White Paper: the chapter on the Home Office', *Public Money* September: 34–44.

McKeown, T. (1979) *The Role of Medicine*, Oxford: Basil Blackwell.

Marsden, D. and Evans, R. (1985) 'Accountable regimes at Featherstone Prison 1981–1984', *Prison Service Journal* April: 4–6.

Matthews, R. (1979) 'Accountable management in the DHSS', *Management Services in Government* 34: 125–32.

Mayston, D. (1985) 'Non-profit performance indicators in the public sector', *Financial Accountability and Management* 1, 1: 51–74.

Merrison, A. (chairman) (1979) *Royal Commission on the National Health Service: Report*, London: HMSO, Cmnd. 7615.

Metcalfe, L. and Richards, S. (1987) *Improving Public Management*, London: Sage.

Monopolies and Mergers Commission (1981) *Severn-Trent Water Authority*, London: HMSO.

Monopolies and Mergers Commission (1985) *British Airports Authority: A Report on the Efficiency and Costs of, and the Service Provided by, the British Airports Authority in its Commercial Activities*, London: HMSO.

Monopolies and Mergers Commission (1986) *Southern Water Authority*, London: HMSO.

Monopolies and Mergers Commission (1987) *British Railways Board: Network South East: A Report on Rail Passenger Services Supplied by the Board in the South East of England*, London: HMSO.

Monopolies and Mergers Commission (1989) *British Railways Board: Provincial: A Report on Rail Passenger Services Supplied by the Board in Great Britain for which the Board's Provincial Sector takes Financial Responsibility*, London: HMSO.

Moodie, M., Mizen, N., Heron, R., and Mackay, B. (1988) *The Business of Service: The Report of the Regional Organization Scrutiny*, London: Department of Social Security.

Morgan, R. (1985) 'Her Majesty's Inspectorate of Prisons', in M. Maguire *et al. Accountability and Prisons: Opening Up a Closed World*, London: Tavistock.

Morgan, R. (1987) *Police*, in M. Parkinson (ed.) *Reshaping Local Government*, Newbury: Policy Journals.

National Audit Office (1986) *The Financial Management Initiative*, London: HMSO, HC 588.

National Audit Office (1988) *Department of Health and Social Security: Quality of Service to the Public*, London: HMSO, HC 451.

National Consumer Council (1986) *Measuring Up: Consumer Assessment of Local Authority Services*, London: NCC.

North East Thames Regional Health Authority (1984) *Responses to DHSS 1985 Package of Performance Indicators*, mimeo.

Pendleton, A. (1988) 'Markets or politics?: the determinants of labour relations in a nationalised industry', *Public Administration* 66, 3: 279–96.

Perrow, C. (1977) 'The Bureaucratic Paradox: the efficient organisation centralizes in order to decentralize', *Organisational Dynamics* Spring: 3–14.

Perry, J. and Kraemer, K. (eds) (1983) *Public Management: Public and Private Perspectives*, Palo Alto: Mayfield.

Pliatzky, L. (1982) *Getting and Spending*, Oxford: Basil Blackwell.

Pollitt, C. (1985) 'Measuring performance: a new system for the National Health Service', *Policy and Politics* 13, 1: 1–15.

Pollitt, C. (1986) 'Beyond the managerial model: the case for broadening performance assessment in government and the public services', *Financial Accountability and Management* 2, 3: 155–70.

Pollitt, C. (1987a) 'Capturing quality? The quality issue in British and American health care policies', *Journal of Public Policy* 7, 1: 71–92.

Pollitt, C. (1987b) 'The politics of performance assessment: lessons for higher education', *Studies in Higher Education* 12, 1: 87–98.

Pollitt, C. (1988) 'Bringing consumers into performance measurement: concepts, consequences and constraints', *Policy and Politics* 16, 2: 77–87.

Pollitt, C. (1989) 'Performance indicators in the public services: the time dimension', paper presented at a seminar at *Brunel University*, 30 January.

Powell, J.E. (1966) *Medicine and Politics*, London: Pitman Medical.

Prescott-Clarke, P., Brooks, T., and Machray, C. (1988) *Focus on Health Care*, London: Royal Institute of Public Administration.

Prime Minister (1970) *The Reorganisation of Central Government*, London: HMSO, Cmnd. 4506.

Prime Minister and Chancellor of the Exchequer (1983) *Financial Management in Government Departments*, London: HMSO, Cmnd. 4506.

Prime Minister and Minister for the Civil Service (1982) *Efficiency and Effectiveness in the Civil Service*, London: HMSO, Cmnd. 8616.

Public Accounts Committee (1981) *Financial Control and Accountability in the National Health Service* (Seventeenth Report, Session 1980–81), London: HMSO, HC 255.

Public Accounts Committee (1985) *Monitoring and Control of the Water Authorities* (Eighteenth Report, Session 1984–85), London: HMSO, HC 249.

Public Accounts Committee (1986) *Efficiency of Nationalised Industries: References to the Monopolies and Mergers Commission* (Fourth Report, Session 1986–87), London: HMSO, HC 26.

Public Accounts Committee (1987) *The Financial Management Initiative*, (Thirteenth Report, Session 1986–87), London: HMSO, HC 61.

Public Accounts Committee (1988) *Quality of Service to the Public at DHSS Local Offices* (Forty-fourth Report, Session 1987–88), London: HMSO, HC 491.

Pugh, D. and Hickson, D. (1976) *Organizational Structure in its Context: The Aston Programme 1*, Aldershot: Gower.

Reiner, R. (1988) 'Keeping the Home Office happy', *Policing* 4, 1: 28–36.

Rivlin, A. (1971) *Systematic Thinking for Social Action*, Washington D.C.: The Brookings Institution.

Rose, R. (1972) 'The market for policy indicators', in A. Shonfield and S. Shaw (eds) *Social Indicators and Social Policy*, London: Heinemann.

Sainsbury, R. (1989) 'The Social Security Chief Adjudication Officer: the first four years', *Public Law* (Summer): 323–41.

Schick, A. (1969) 'Systems politics and systems budgeting', *Public Administrative Review* 29, 2: 137-51.

Schultze, C. (1968) *The Politics and Economics of Public Spending*, Washington D.C.: The Brookings Institution.

Secretary of State for Health (1989) *Working for Patients*, London: HMSO, Cmnd. 555.

Select Committee on Nationalised Industries (1968) *Ministerial Control of the Nationalised Industries* (First Report, Session 1967–68), London: HMSO, HC 371 (3 volumes).

Select Committee on Procedure (1969) *Scrutiny of Public Expenditure and Administration* (First Report, Session 1968–69), London: HMSO, HC 410.

Self, P. (1975) *Econocrats and the Policy Process*, London: Macmillan.

Sinclair, I. and Miller, C. (1984) *Measures of Effectiveness and Efficiency*, London: Home Office Research and Planning Unit.

Skinner, P., Riley, D., and Thomas, E. (1988) 'Use and abuse of performance indicators', *British Medical Journal* 297, 12 November: 1256–9.

Social Services Committee (1980) *The Government's White Papers on Public Expenditure: The Social Services* (Third Report, Session 1979–80), London: HMSO, HC 702-1.

Stowe, K. (1989) *On Caring for the National Health*, London: The Nuffield Provincial Hospitals Trust.

Thomas, H. (1968) *Crisis in the Civil Service*, London: Anthony Blond.

Thomas, K. (1982) 'Framework for branch performance evaluation', *Journal of Retail Banking* 4, 1: 24–34.

Train, C. (1985) 'Management accountability in the prison service', in M. Maguire *et al. Accountability and Prisons: Opening Up a Closed World*, London: Tavistock.

Treasury and Civil Service Committee (1982) *Efficiency and Effectiveness in the Civil Service* (Third Report, Session 1981–82), London: HMSO, HC 236–1.

Treasury and Civil Service Committee (1988) *Civil Service Management Reform: The Next Steps* (Eighth Report, Session 1987–88), London: HMSO, HC 494–1.

Treasury and Civil Service Committee (1990) *Progress in the Next Steps Initiative (Eighth Report, Session 1989–90), London: HMSO, HC 481.*

Universities Funding Council (1989) *Research Selectivity Exercise 1989: The Outcome*, Circular Letter 27/89, London.

US Department of Health, Education, and Welfare (1969) *Towards a Social Report*, Washington D.C.: US Government Printing Office.

Vickers, G. (1965) *The Art of Judgement*, London: Chapman and Hall.

Vickers, J. and Yarrow, G. (1988) *Privatization: An Economic Analysis*, Cambridge, Mass.: MIT Press.

Walton, R. (1975) 'MBO in the regional organization of the DHSS', *Management Services in Government* 30, 2: 93–109.

Water Authorities Association (1986) *Waterfacts*, London.

Weatheritt, M. (1986) *Innovations in Policing*, London: Croom Helm (with Police Foundation).

Webber, R. and Craig, J. (1976) *Which Local Authorities are Alike?*, London: HMSO.

Wildavsky, A. (1979) *Speaking Truth to Power: The Art and Craft of Policy Analysis*, Boston: Little, Brown, and Company.

Williams, A. (1967) *Output Budgeting and the Contribution of Micro-economics to Efficiency in Government*, London: HMSO.

Woodward, S. (1986) 'Performance indicators and management performance in nationalised industries', *Public Administration* 64, 3: 303–17.

Wright, M. (1977) 'Public expenditure in Britain: the crisis of control', *Public Administration* 55, 2: 143–69.

Zuboff, S. (1988) *In the Age of the Smart Machine*, New York: Basic Books.

Name index

Abel-Smith, B. 105
Aldrich, H. 27

Banks, G.T. 9
Barratt, R. 60
Beard, W. 44
Beeching, Lord 142
Bevan, Aneurin 103
Birch, R. 93, 95, 97
Bramley, G. 47
Brophy, Jim 160, 161, 162, 163, 164
Buswell, D. 134
Butler, T. 56
Butt, H. 36

Caines, K. 23
Carter, N. 20, 35, 43, 181, 182
Cartwright, A. 176
Cave, M. 43, 44
Chadwick, Edwin 13
Challis, L. 7
Chaplin, B. 82
Christian, J. 54
Clarke, P. 39
Clarke, R. 79
Clegg, S. 27
Collins, K. 55
Cornish, D. 79
Craig, J. 47
Crick, B. 6
Cubbon, Sir Brian 55
Cyert, J. 33

Day, P. 32, 64, 104, 111, 117, 149,
    150, 152, 175, 180

Dunbar, I. 80, 81, 82, 84
Dunkerley, D. 27
Dunleavy, P. 27
Dunsire, A. 27, 29

Evans, R. 82, 83

Ferner, A. 144
Flynn, A. 20 37, 38, 39
Flynn, N. 36, 48
Fowler, Norman 106
Fulton, Lord 10

Garrett, J. 45, 91
Goldman, H. 79
Gray, J. 32
Gretton, J. 57
Guillebaud, C. 104

Harrison, A. 57
Heclo, H. 10
Heseltine, Michael 18
Hickson, D. 27
Hill, M. 47
Hitch, Charles 7
Hood, C. 27
Hopkins, A. 177
Hopwood, A. 28

Jackson, A. 23
Jackson, P. 37, 38, 43, 44
Jenkin, Patrick 106
Jenkins, K. 23, 179
Jenkins, L. 113, 114
Jesson, D. 32

Johnson, President 7, 15
Jones, S. 55
Jowett, P. 26
Joyce, M. 26, 36, 37, 48

Kanter, R. 42
King, A. 6
King, R. 82
Klein, R. 9, 10, 32, 64, 104, 105, 106, 111, 117, 149, 150, 152, 175, 180
Körner, Edith 106
Kraemer, K. 29

Levitt, M. 26, 36, 37, 48
Lord, R. 87

McKeown, T. 103
McNamara, Robert 7
Major, John 179
March, J. 33
Marsden, D. 82
Matthews, R. 91
Maxwell, R. 177
Mayston, D. 139
Merrison, A. 102, 103
Metcalfe, L. 6, 17
Middleton, Sir Peter 23, 38
Miller, C. 53, 58
Moodie, M. 96
Morgan, R. 80, 81, 83
Moser, Claus 15

Nairne, Sir Patrick 106, 107, 109
Newman, Sir Kenneth 57
Newton, Tony 99

Olson, Mancur 15

Palmer, A. 37, 38
Palmer, B. 36
Pendleton, A. 141, 142, 144
Perrow, C. 19, 170, 179
Perry, J. 29
Pliatzky, L. 16
Pollitt, C. 26, 38, 39, 40, 41, 42, 43, 45, 107, 116, 172
Powell, J.E. 105, 113
Prescott-Clarke, P. 176
Pugh, D. 27

Rayner, Sir Derek 16, 17, 19, 67
Reiner, R. 57
Richards, S. 6, 17
Rivlin, Alice 12–13, 15, 40
Rose, Richard 16, 179
Rothwell, M. 26

Sainsbury, R. 99
Schick, A. 7–9
Schultze, C. 7
Self, P. 13
Shonfield, Andrew 15
Silverman, E. 55
Sinclair, I. 53, 58
Skinner, P. 113
Stowe, K. 106
Summers, D. 42

Thatcher, Margaret 10, 16, 17, 179
Thomas, H. 6
Thomas, K. 127, 128
Train, C. 82

Vickers, G. 28
Vickers, J. 150, 158, 159

Walton, R. 91
Weatheritt, M. 54
Webber, R. 47
Wildavsky, A. 9, 10
Williams, A. 13
Woodward, S. 139
Wright, M. 16

Yarrow, G. 150, 158, 159
Yates, John 107
Young, Lord 49

Zuboff, S. 181

Subject index

academic research 44, 49–50
acceptability of PIs and performance measurement 45, 173; British Rail 143, 145; courts 76; NHS 108, 113, 116; police 62–3; prisons 86, Social Security 91, 101; water industry 152, 154
acceptable performance *see* standards
accountability of organisations 10, 19, 30–1, 35, 138–40, 166, 170, 173, 180, 181, 182; BAA 159; British Rail 140, 143; courts 66; government 19, 165–7, 182–3; NHS 103, 104, 106, 107, 109, 115, 117; police 52, 53, 64, 171; prisons 79, 85; to the public 19–20, 31, 89–90; Social Security 89, 91, 171; water industry 150
accountancy 26, 28
accuracy *see* reliability
Acorn system 122
activity analysis 58
activity measurement 14, 20–1, 36, 166; courts 67, 70; NHS 116; police 58–60, 64; prisons 82, 83, 84, 85, 87; *see also* outputs
administrative tribunals 40
agencies 20, 23, 26, 28, 29, 35, 48, 170, 179; NHS as 103, 104; Social Security as 89, 96, 101, 178; *see also* branches
aims: prisons 82; water industry 151–2
airports *see* BAA plc
Airports Act (1986) 160
ambiguity: of government's objectives

concerning PIs 165; of PIs 49, 50, 166
Aston Group 27
Audit Commission 26, 30, 32, 36, 37, 39, 47, 115
authority 33, 35, 171–2; BAA 159; British Rail 140; NHS 170; police 171; prisons 78; Social Security 90; *see also* control
autonomy 35, 170, 171, 172; BAA 159; commerce 123; courts 76; NHS 104, 176, 178; police 53, 63; prisons 78, 86, 171; Social Security 90, water industry 150; *see also* control

BAA plc 26, 30, 34, 138, 139, 158–64; design and use of PIs in 159–64, 172
bailiffs 71, 73
banks 3, 28, 30, 34, 48, 125–35, 172; *see also* financial institutions
Bexley Council 46
bonuses *see* performance related pay
boundedness of PIs *see* quantity of PIs
branches 26, 35, 43, 118, 137, 172; financial institutions 28, 126, 127–31, 132; managers *see* managers; shops 120, 124, 125; *see also* agencies
British Airports Authority *see* BAA plc
British Airways 141
British Rail 29, 30, 31, 34, 138, 139, 140–9, 172; design and use of PIs

29, 142–9, 168; flexible rostering dispute 144; Productivity Steering Group 143
British Telecom 30, 31, 180
budgetary systems 13
budgeting, output *see* output budgeting
budgets: BR 143, 144; NHS 105; police 81, 88
building societies 28, 34, 48, 125–35; *see also* financial institutions
Building Societies Act (1986) 127
business: government and 17, 19; *see also* consumerism
Business of Service, The 96

Cabinet Office 166
Callaghan Administration 54
Care in Action 106
case studies 2–4, 21, 26, 51, 167–78; *see also individual organisations*
Central Statistical Office 15
Central Transport Consultative (CTCC) 140, 141, 142, 146, 147, 148
centralisation: BAA 159; of government activities 19, 58, 106, 107, 108, 117, 170, 179; private sector 119, 121, 122, 125, 127, 129, 130, 132–3, 137; *see also* control; decentralisation
Challenge of the 80s 143
Chancellor of the Exchequer 10
Chartered Institute of Public Finance and Accountancy (CIPFA) 26, 36, 47, 63
Chessington Computer Centre 21
CIPFA *see* Chartered Institute of Public Finance and Accountancy
Circuit Objectives 67
citation circles 44, 49
Citibank 134
citizens advice bureaux 89
Civil Aviation Authority 160
civil service 1, 6, 10, 13, 17, 20, 182; Financial Management Initiative *see* Financial Management Initiative; Next Steps Initiative *see* Next Steps Initiative; *see also* government departments
cluster analysis 47, 60, 86, 87, 98, 115

Committee of Enquiry into the Cost of the National Health Service 104
Comparing Health Authorities 110
comparison between organisations 46–8; BAA 160, 161; BR 143, 144; courts 74; NHS 111, 114–16; police 60–1; prisons 84, 86, 87; private sector 121, 122, 130, 131–2; Social Security 95, 98; water industry 152
competition and organisations 29–30, 41, 174; courts 66; nationalised industries 139, 141, 148, 150, 159; private sector 118, 120, 121–2, 126, 127, 131, 133, 135; Social Security 89
complaints 40, 41, 50, 59, 60, 75, 95, 99, 120, 122–3, 125, 134, 136, 137, 140, 148, 153, 154, 157, 162, 174; *see also* consumers; quality of service
complexity of organisations 32–3, 44, 181; individual 53, 66, 72, 78, 90, 102, 118, 127, 140–1, 150, 159, 170, 171, 172
comprehensibility of PIs 182
computerisation 45; NHS 108, 111; police 63; prisons 86; *see also* information, information systems; statistics
Conservative Administrations 1, 5, 10, 16–17, 30; and nationalised industries 139, 140, 141, 143, 144, 149, 151, 152, 155, 157, 158, 159, 160, 163; and NHS 105–6, 175; and police 54–5; and prisons 79–80; and Social Security 90, 95
Conservative Central Office 16
consumer surveys 64, 99–100, 134, 157, 163, 174, 176, 178
consumerism 96, 101, 174–6
consumers 30, 41, 42, 43, 174–8, 182; and BAA 163, 172; and BR 148; and courts 75; and NHS 116, 175; and police 64, 175; and prisons 84, 175; and private sector 122, 123, 133–5, 136; and Social Security 96, 99–101; and water industry 157, 158, 172; *see also* complaints; quality of service

Contributions Unit 89
control: BAA 160; nationalised
  industries 138–40, 141, 156; NHS
  106, 107, 109, 110, 112, 113, 117,
  170; police 53, 58, 63, 64–5;
  prisons 77, 78, 84–5; private sector
  119, 121, 122, 125, 127, 129, 130,
  132–3, 137; water industry 150
control, political 6, 10, 19, 35, 173;
  PIs as tools of 2, 42, 43, 45, 173,
  179, 180, 181; in United States
  7–9; *see also* accountability
corporate plans 145, 147, 153
cost–benefit analysis 13, 14
cost centres 47, 67, 82
costs 5, 21, 37, 39; BAA 161, 163; BR
  142, 145; courts 65, 67, 70, 71–2;
  NHS 106, 116; police 54–5, 58, 59,
  60; prisons 80, 81–2, 86–8; private
  sector 128, 136; Social Security 91,
  98; water industry 151, 152, 155,
  158; *see also* inputs; resources
County Courts 65, 66, 68, 70–2
Court of Appeal 65
courts 34, 65–77; design and use of
  PIs in 67–77, 171
crime levels 32, 33, 46, 54
criminal justice system *see* courts;
  police; prisons
Criminal Statistics 56, 57
Crown Courts 65, 66, 68, 69, 70, 71,
  73, 74, 75, 76
customer profiles 130
customers *see* consumers
Customs and Excise 48

decentralisation 1, 2, 19, 23, 106, 109,
  166, 170, 178, 179, 180, 182; *see
  also* centralisation; control
decision making 7, 8–9, 111
definition of PIs 35–41
delegation 11, 103, 104; *see also*
  control; decentralisation
Department of Education and
  Science 9, 10, 14, 15, 35, 43
Department of Health (1989–) 103,
  107, 111, 114–15, 169, 176
Department of Health and Social
  Security 9, 18, 45, 50, 106, 107,
  108, 109, 110, 115

Department of Social Security (1989–)
  89, 96, 99, 179
Department of the Environment 18,
  20, 150, 151, 153, 155; Code of
  Practice 19
Department of Transport 145, 158
descriptive PIs 49–50, 137, 168, 169;
  BR 144; courts 70; financial
  institutions 130; NHS 115; prisons
  86; Social Security 98; water
  industry 153
design of PIs 26, 42, 51, 165, 167–8,
  171, 183; *see also individual
  organisations*
Director-General of Water Services
  158
disaggregation/aggregation of figures
  43, 56, 80, 81, 84, 98, 121, 129,
  132–3, 134, 136, 145, 146, 147,
  149, 152, 153, 161
distribution of power 8
Drinking Water Inspectorate 158
Driver and Vehicle Licensing Centre 21
Driving Standards Agency 180

economics, economists: influence on
  techniques of government 13–15,
  26
Economist, The 133, 134, 158
economy 30, 35, 37, 39; *see also* costs
education 14, 32, 35, 43, 47, 48
effectiveness of PIs 43–5
effectiveness of service 18, 19, 21, 22,
  30, 35, 37, 38–9, 41, 165; BR 144,
  149; courts 69, 74–5, 76; NHS
  106; police 55, 57, 64; prisons 79,
  84; private sector 119, 125, 127;
  Social Security 90, 92, 99; water
  industry 153, 154
efficacy 39
efficiency 1, 11, 12, 17, 18, 19, 21, 26,
  30, 35, 37–8, 39, 40, 42, 166, 180,
  181, 183; BAA 160, 161; courts
  65, 68, 69, 71–2, 74, 76;
  nationalised industries 139, 143,
  144; NHS 105, 106, 107, 108, 112;
  police 54, 55, 56, 57, 59, 64;
  prisons 80-1; private sector 119,
  122, 125, 135; Social Security 98;
  water industry 151, 152, 158

efficiency strategy 6
Efficiency Unit 16–17, 23, 179
Electricity Council 49
electricity industry 49
electronic point of sale data capture 119
environment: concern about 158
Environment Committee 157
environmental factors affecting organisations 32, 54, 57, 79, 90, 97, 98, 101, 120, 122, 127, 142, 156–7
equity 39–40, 183; access to NHS 102, 108, 116
ethics and government methods 13–14
European Community 151, 154, 155, 158
evaluation 1–2, 19
evaluation, self- *see* self-evaluation
Expenditure Committee 12

Famibank 134
Family Practitioner Committees 103, 107
financial institutions: deregulation in 1980s 126, 133; technological innovations 126; *see also* banks; building societies
financial management in government *see* Financial Management Initiative
Financial Management Initiative 1982 (FMI) 2, 5–6, 7, 10, 11, 17, 18, 20, 21, 22, 23, 37, 43, 44, 165, 166, 178, 179, 182; and individual organisations 55, 56, 58, 64, 67, 76, 80, 81, 82, 91, 95, 107
financial PIs 29, 120, 128–9, 136, 139, 142, 143, 149, 151, 152, 160, 162; *see also* profit
flexibility: of data 85–6, 94; in financial institutions 132
friendly societies 127
Fulton Committee on the Civil Service 10, 11, 19, 23, 31, 91, 179

General Municipal Boilermakers and Allied Trades Union 109
government 6; culture of 1, 2, 17, 107, 166; finance *see* public expenditure; management of 1–2, 5–24, 165–7, 178–83
government departments 2, 5, 12, 20, 48, 49, 91, 107, 170; *see also* individual departments
green issues 158
Guardian, The 158

Hansard 47
Health Service Indicators Group 109, 116
Heath Administration 10, 95
Her Majesty's Stationery Office 21, 29
Her Majesty's Treasury 5, 9, 10, 11, 16, 20, 21–2, 23, 30, 67, 68, 70, 72, 91, 166; Centre for Administrative Studies 13; Cmnd Paper 1009 52, 56, 57, 69, 71, 77, 81; Cmnd Paper 1013 113; Cmnd Paper 1014 92, 93, 100; model of PIs 36, 37; Public Expenditure White Paper *see* Public Expenditure White Paper
heterogeneity 32, 44, 48, 53, 78, 90, 102, 118, 127, 150, 159, 170, 171, 172, 181
High Street retailers 34, 118–25, 174, 177
Home Office, Home Secretary 53, 54, 56, 57, 59–65 *passim*, 80, 82; Circular 114/1983 55–6, 57, 58, 65; Circular 55/1984 82, 83; Circular 35/1989 65
Home Office/Inspectorate working group on activity measures (1986) 59
homogeneity of courts 66
House of Commons 11–12, 106; *see also* Parliament
House of Commons Committee of Public Accounts *see* Public Accounts Committee
housing 14

impact *see* outcome
incentives: staff 48; to use PIs 45–6; *see also* performance related pay
Independent, The 49, 155, 157
individual appraisal 42, 45, 131, 163

information, information systems:
accuracy *see* reliability; BR 144,
148; commerce 120, 121, 122, 123,
124; courts 72, 73, 76;
disaggregation/ aggregation of
figures *see* disaggregation/
aggregation of figures; Expenditure Committee and 12; financial
institutions 128, 130, 132; NHS
104, 105, 106, 107, 109, 111, 112,
113; police 55, 63, 65; prisons 79,
80–1, 83–8; Social Security 91, 94,
101; water industry 157; *see also*
statistics
information technology 1, 44, 45, 46,
110, 111, 180, 181; *see also*
computerisation
Information Technology Services
Agency 89
Inland Revenue 41, 48, 91
inputs 17, 23, 33, 35–6, 37, 48;
individual organisations 54, 82, 84,
91, 111, 142, 143, 150, 159; *see
also* resources
Inspectorate of Constabulary 53, 56,
58, 59, 60, 61, 62, 63, 64
Inspectorate of Pollution 158
InterCity 140, 141, 145, 146, 147, 148
interdependence in organisations *see*
performance ownership
intermediate output *see* outputs
international agreements on airlines 160
international water standards 151,
154, 155, 158

Joint Consultative Committee of the
three Police Staff Associations in
England and Wales 56, 58, 61, 63, 65
Judicial Statistics 67
Jupiter TVhire 34, 118, 135–7

Kent police 63
King's College Hospital, London,
Department of Trauma and
Orthopaedics 113

Labour Administrations 54, 139
league tables 47, 74, 95, 121, 144
life insurance companies 48
Lloyds Bank Economic Bulletin 126

local authorities 19, 30, 53, 89, 115,
158
local education authorities 35, 43
Lord Chancellor's Department *see*
courts

management: skill and introduction
of PIs 45–6; styles of, and uses of
PIs 42, 50, 181
Management by Objectives 45, 91
management consultants 81
Management Information System for
Ministers (MINIS) 18, 44
management strategy: PIs as part of
2, 21, 42, 63, 84–5, 87, 107, 110,
115, 117, 157, 163, 167, 173, 181,
182
management structure: BAA 159;
BR 140–1; commerce 119–21,
133; courts 65, 72–7; financial
institutions 127, 128; Jupiter
TVhire 136; NHS 103–4; police
55, 58, 63; prisons 77, 80–8; Social
Security 90; water industry 150,
155–6
managerial rationalism 7
managers, private sector 137, 172;
commerce 119, 120–1, 122, 123;
financial institutions 127, 128, 129,
130, 131, 133
managers, public sector: BAA 163;
and consumer 41; and
performance measures 42
*Manpower, Effectiveness and
Efficiency in the Police Service* 55
market ideology *see also* consumerism
May Committee of Inquiry (1979) 80,
81, 82
media: and courts 66; and prisons
178; and Social Security 90
Metropolitan Police 53, 57
MINIS *see* Management Information
System for Ministers
Ministers 6, 11, 17, 19, 21, 94, 138,
182; *see also individual ministers*
Ministry of Defence 9, 20
models of PIs 35–40
monopolies, monopoly 30, 41, 52, 66,
77, 89, 126, 139, 172, 173, 182; *see
also individual organisations*

Monopolies and Mergers
  Commission 140, 145, 146, 152,
  159, 160, 162, 163
MPs and PIs 182–3

National Audit Office (NAO) 22, 72,
  73, 74, 76, 81, 89, 93, 94, 95, 100,
  178
National Consumer Council 41, 43
National Farmers Union 157
National Health Service 3, 29, 31–2,
  33, 34, 89, 90, 102–17, 123;
  contract system 176, 177, 178,
  180; design and use of PIs in 46,
  50, 104–17, 168, 169, 170, 171,
  173, 175, 176, 177–8, 180, 181
National Health Service and
  Community Care Act (1990) 104
National Rivers Authority 31, 158
National Westminster Bank 133
nationalised industries *see* public
  utilities
Nationalised Industries White Paper
  (1978) 30–1, 139, 143, 151, 159
Naval Aircraft Repair Organisation 21
negative PIs *see* proscriptive PIs
Netherlands: rail service 149
Network SouthEast 140, 141, 145–6,
  148
Next Steps Initiative 23, 24, 179–80
North East Thames Regional Health
  Authority 40

objectives 5, 12, 13, 18, 19, 21, 33, 35,
  37, 38, 39, 49, 167, 169, 170, 182;
  agencies 179; BAA 159, 161;
  courts 67–70, 72, 73, 74–7;
  financial institutions 130, 131; of
  government in introducing PIs
  165–6; NHS 105, 106; police 54,
  55, 60, 62; prisons 78–9, 82; Social
  Security 90, 101; water industry
  150, 153, 155
objectives, multiple 14, 22, 25, 28, 32,
  33, 46, 175, 181; BR 141–2; of
  government 165, 180; NHS 102,
  104; police 53–4; prisons 78–9
Observer, The 155
Office of Telecommunications 15
Oftel *see* Office of Telecommunications

ombudsmen 40
operational evaluation in financial
  institutions 128, 129
organisations: characteristics 3,
  27–35, 41, 51, 77, 167, 170–3,
  177–8 *see also individual
  characteristics*; culture of 45;
  management of *see* management;
  rate of evolvement of PIs 21, 172–3
outcome 14, 28, 33, 36–7, 166, 177,
  181; BAA 159; BR 142, 145;
  commerce 118; courts 66; NHS
  103, 109, 114; police 53, 54; water
  industry 150
output budgeting, 7, 12, 13–15; *see
  also* planning, programming,
  budgeting (PPB) system
outputs 5, 9, 11, 12, 13, 14, 17, 18, 19,
  20, 28, 35–9, 166, 174, 176, 182;
  BAA 159; BR 142, 143;
  commerce 118, 122; courts 72;
  NHS 105, 111, 112; police 53, 54,
  58, 59, 60, 64; prisons 82, 87;
  Social Security 90, 91, 92, 101;
  water industry 152; *see also*
  throughput
overload 6
ownership of organisations and PIs
  29; *see also* public/private divide
ownership of performance *see*
  performance ownership

PAC *see* Public Accounts Committee
Parliament 6, 10, 11, 12, 17, 19, 103,
  106, 138, 165, 182–3; and BR 140;
  and courts 66; and water industry
  150
parliamentary questions 40, 94, 140
parliamentary reports 11–12, 13, 18,
  182
performance: definition of
  dimensions of 2
performance measurement 1–2,
  20–4; background to 5–20; future
  prospects 182–3; literature 26,
  36–41, 50; problems 21–2, 50, 51;
  vocabulary 7, 17, 26, 36–41; *for
  individual organisations see
  organisation*
performance ownership 31, 32–3, 43,

46, 166, 170, 171, 172; BAA 159, 162; courts 66–7; NHS 31–2; police 54; prisons 79, 83; private sector 119, 124, 127, 136; Social Security 93; water industry 156

performance related pay 42, 43, 45, 131, 136, 142, 157–8, 163–4

planning, programming, budgeting (PPB) system 7–9, 12, 14, 15, 16, 179; police 54; *see also* output budgeting

Plowden Report 10

police 33, 34, 52–65; culture of 63–4; design and use of PIs 29, 52, 54–65, 168, 169, 170–1, 175; Unit Beat Policing 54

Police Foundation 65

Policing by Objectives (PBO) 55–6, 63

politicians 41, 42; *see also* Parliament

Post Office 29

prescriptive PIs 49, 50, 115, 137, 149, 155, 168–9, 173, 174, 177

Prime Minister 9, 16, 17, 20, 169–70, 179

priorities: police 55, 56

Prison Board 82

Prison Department 77, 82

Prison Officers Association 81

Prison Statistics 80

prisons 34, 77–88; 'Fresh Start' agreement 81, 87, 88; performance measurement 46, 77, 79–88, 169, 171, 178; Strangeways riot (1990) 78

private detective agencies 52

private sector 2, 3, 27, 28, 29, 30, 31, 48, 51, 118–37, 168, 169, 170, 172, 173, 174, 175–6; use of non-profit PIs 137

private security police industry 52

privatisation 180, 182; BAA 158, 159; water 138 157, 158

process politics 8–9

processes 36, 54, 87, 99, 118, 166, 174, 176, 177, 181

productivity 63, 81, 98, 116, 132, 139, 142, 143, 144, 145, 149, 157, 163

professionalism, professionals 35, 41, 42, 58, 60, 61, 65, 75, 104, 113, 127, 150, 170, 178

profit 27–8, 118–19, 128, 131, 135, 137, 160, 169, 170, 171, 174

Programme Analysis and Review (PAR) 10, 16, 179

proscriptive PIs 49, 169, 174, 177; individual organisations 80, 85, 87, 93, 101, 122, 125, 137, 155, 163

Provincial sector of British Rail 140, 145, 146

public: accountability to 19–20, 31, 89–90; *see also* consumers

Public Accounts Committee (PAC) 22, 23, 38, 55, 95, 96, 98, 100, 106, 145, 152, 153, 165

public expenditure 10–13, 16, 17, 19, 20, 23, 30, 55, 68, 116, 151, 166, 180

Public Expenditure White Paper 10, 20, 21, 56, 67, 70, 80, 100, 182; for 1990 52, 56, 57, 69, 71, 72, 77, 81, 92, 93, 100, 112, 113

public limited companies 127

Public Money 81

public opinion surveys 58

public/private divide 3, 25, 27, 29, 30, 31, 51, 168, 169, 173

public sector 2, 3, 27, 29, 35, 176; and competition 30 *see also* competition; and economy 37; and equity 39–40; and performance measurement 22–4, 42–3, 44, 49, 50, 168, 169–70, 173, 177, 178; *see also* public services; public utilities

Public Service Obligation (PSO) grants 141, 145

public services 2, 41, 174–5; *see also* individual organisations

public utilities 29, 138–64, 171–2, 173, 174, 182; social obligations 141; *see also individual organisations*

quality of service 25, 37, 40–1, 174–8; BAA 160, 161, 162–3; BR 142, 144, 145–9; courts 75; nationalised industries 31, 139; NHS 102, 109, 116; police 64; prisons 80, 84; private sector 121, 123, 125, 133; Social Security 91, 95, 96, 99–101; water industry 151–8; *see also* complaints; standards quantity of

PIs 44, 167, 168, 171, 181–2; NHS 108, 110; police 63; prisons 85; private sector 124, 125, 137; railways 145, 149; Social Security 101, 171

railways *see* British Rail
Rand Corporation 7
reliability of information and PIs 44; NHS 113; prisons 86; private sector 125, 130; Social Security 93, 94, 98
Reorganisation of Central Government, The 9–10
Report of HM Inspector of Constabulary 56
Resettlement Agency 89
resources 36, 173, 175, 176, 180, 181; individual organisations 55, 69, 73, 74, 76, 98, 108, 111, 112, 116, 149; *see also* inputs
responsibility *see* accountability
Royal College of Surgeons 109
Royal Commission on Sewerage Disposal (1912) 151
Royal Commission on the National Health Service (1979) 102, 103

Secretary of State for Health 103, 181, 182
Secretary of State for the Environment 150, 158
Secretary of State for Transport 145, 147
Secretary of State for Wales 150
Select Committee on Nationalised Industries (1968) 138–9
self-evaluation: PIs and organisational 2, 21, 42, 87, 107, 110, 115, 117, 157, 163, 167, 173, 181, 182
Sense of Direction, A (Dunbar) 80, 81, 82, 84
Severn-Trent water region 157–8
shops *see* High Street retailers; supermarkets
social change 1
social indicators 15–16
Social Science Research Council 15
Social Security 34, 40, 65, 66, 89–101, 134; design and use of PIs 3, 32, 38, 41, 46, 91–101, 171, 178
Social Security White Paper 93–4
Social Services Committee 106
Social Trends 15
South West Water 157
Southern Water Authority 152
staff 102, 142, 150, 156, 171; absenteeism 123, 132, 137; incentives 45, 48 *see also* performance related pay; management of 123–4, 125, 131, 132, 134; and PIs 42, 87, *see also* acceptability of PIs and performance measurement
standards 46, 49, 50, 51, 169, 172, 176, 180; individual organisations 92, 100, 101, 105, 123, 125, 138, 144, 146, 147, 149, 151, 154, 155, 158, 161
state *see* government
'Statement of the Functions of Prison Department Establishments' 82
'Statement of the Tasks of the Prison Service' 82
statistics 14, 16, 20–1; BR 142; commerce 122, 124; courts 67; NHS 107, 110, 115, 116, 173; police 56–7, 58, 59–65
strategic planning 121, 148
subsidies, rail 141, 145
supermarkets 3, 28, 34, 118–25, 133, 134, 171, 172, 174, 175, 177, 181
systems approach to performance measurement 7–10, 12, 17

takeovers 28, 119
targets 19, 20, 38, 39, 46, 49, 50, 169, 181; agencies 179–80; courts 67, 68, 69, 71, 72–3, 75, 76, 77; nationalised industries 141–5 *passim*, 147, 149, 151–2, 162–3; NHS 111, 112, 115, 176, 180; police 63; prisons 84; private sector 120, 121, 122, 124, 125, 130, 136, 137; Social Security 91, 95, 96–8, 101, 171, 178
Thatcher Administration *see* Conservative Administrations
throughput 36, 69, 72, 74–5, 98, 152; *see also* outputs

time-and-motion studies 45
time-series comparisons 46–7, 50, 60,
  84, 130, 136, 152, 153, 155, 161
timeliness of information 44, 167,
  168, 171, 176, 182; BAA 163; BR
  148; courts 73; NHS 111, 112,
  116–17; police 60–1; prisons 85;
  private sector 122, 124, 134,
  136–7; Social Security 101, 171;
  water industry 154, 157
trade unions 35, 45, 90, 91, 95
trading status of organisations 29, 30,
  171–2, 173; individual
  organisations 52, 66, 77, 89, 102,
  139, 159
transport industry 139, 141, 148; *see
  also* BAA plc; British Rail
Treasury *see* Her Majesty's Treasury
Treasury and Civil Service Committee
  (1982) 18–19, 23, 37–8, 179

uncertainty in organisations 32, 33,
  173, 181; individual organisations
  53, 54, 66, 78–9, 88, 90, 103, 118,
  141–2, 150, 159, 166, 170, 171, 172
United States 7–9, 12, 40;
  Department of Defense 7;

Department of Health, Education

and Welfare 15
universities 47; *see also* academic
  research
Universities Funding Council 47
University of Birmingham Health
  Services Management Unit 107
uses of PIs 2, 42–51, 167, 168–70,
  182; *see also individual
  organisations*; descriptive PIs;
  prescriptive PIs; proscriptive PIs

value for money 1, 16, 18, 20, 60, 63,
  80, 108, 116, 166
Vehicle Inspectorate 21

Water Acts: 1945 151; 1973 151;
  1983 150
Water Authorities Association 150,
  151, 152, 156
water industry 34, 136, 138, 139,
  149–58, 180; design and use of PIs
  in 31, 49, 150–8, 172, 177
White Paper on Nationalised Industries
  (1978) 30–1, 139, 143, 151, 159
work process 35
work study 142
workforce *see* staff
workload analysis 58
World Health Organisation 151